Table of Contents

3

Introduction

Are you looking for an easy way to cook healthy meals in the comfort of your own home? Are you searching for simple kitchen tools that will help you prepare some rich and delicious dishes for you and your loved ones? Well, if that's the case, then this is the best guide you could use.

This cooking guide presents to you the best and most innovative cooking tool available these days. We're talking about the instant pot. This original and useful pot has gained so many fans all over the world due to the fact that it's so easy to use and because it can help you cook so many delicious meals. You can prepare easy breakfasts, lunch dishes, snacks, appetizers, side dishes, fish and seafood, meat, poultry, vegetable and dessert recipes instant pot

This brings us to the second part of this guide. This journal focuses on using the instant pot to make the best Ketogenic dishes. The Ketogenic diet is much more than a simple weight loss program. It's a lifestyle that will improve your health and the way you look.

This low-carb and high-fat diet will get your body to a state of ketosis. The diet help you produce more ketones and therefore it will improve your metabolism and your energy levels.

The Ketogenic diet will show its multiple benefits in a matter of minutes and it will help you look and feel better.

All you need to do now is to get your hands on a copy of this great recipes collection because it brings you the best Ketogenic meals made in an instant pot.

You will enjoy each of these great dishes.

So, let's start this culinary trip right away. Have fun cooking in your instant pot and enjoy the multiple benefits of the Ketogenic diet.

Ketogenic Instant Pot Breakfast Recipes

Soft Eggs and Avocado Mix
Preparation time: 5 minutes | Cooking time: 3 minutes | Servings: 2

Ingredients:

- 2 cups water
- 4 eggs
- 1 avocado, peeled and cubed
- 1 tomato, cubed
- 2 teaspoons avocado oil
- A pinch of salt and black pepper
- 1 teaspoon balsamic vinegar

Directions:

Put the water in the instant pot, add the steamer basket, add the eggs inside, put the lid on and cook on Low for 3 minutes. Release the pressure fast for 5 minutes, cool the eggs down, peel, cut them into quarters and put them in a bowl. Add the avocado and the rest of the ingredients, toss a bit, divide between plates and serve.

Nutrition: calories 170, fat 14.7, fiber 3.2, carbs 5.5, protein 6

Blackberry Muffins
Preparation time: 10 minutes | Cooking time: 20 minutes | Servings: 4

Ingredients:

- 1 and ½ tablespoons flaxseed meal
- ½ cup coconut flour
- 4 tablespoons swerve
- 1 teaspoon baking powder
- ½ cup almond milk
- ¼ teaspoon baking soda
- 2 eggs, whisked
- 1 and ½ tablespoons ghee, melted
- 1 teaspoon vanilla extract
- ½ cup blackberries
- 1 cup water

Directions:

In a bowl, combine the flaxmeal with the flour, swerve and the rest of the ingredients except the water and whisk well. Divide this into a muffin pan. Put the water in the instant pot, add the steamer basket, put the muffin pan inside, put the lid on and cook on High for 20 minutes. Release the pressure naturally for 10 minutes, cool the muffins down and serve for breakfast.

Nutrition: calories 112, fat 9.1, fiber 1.1, carbs 4.2, protein 4.8

Spinach Frittata

Preparation time: 10 minutes | Cooking time: 10 minutes | Servings: 4

Ingredients:

- 6 eggs, whisked
- 1 cup baby spinach
- 1 spring onion, minced
- ½ teaspoon garlic powder
- A pinch of salt and black pepper
- 1 cup water
- Cooking spray

Directions:

In a bowl, combine the eggs with the spinach and the rest of the ingredients except the water and the cooking spray and whisk well. Grease a pan with the cooking spray and pour the frittata mix inside. Put the water in the instant pot, add the trivet, put the pan inside, put the lid on and cook on High for 10 minutes. Release the pressure naturally for 10 minutes, divide the frittata between plates and serve.

Nutrition: calories 103, fat 6.4, fiber 1.1, carbs 2.5, protein 8.4

Broccoli Casserole

Preparation time: 10 minutes | Cooking time: 40 minutes | Servings: 4

Ingredients:

- 3 broccoli stalks, grated
- 2 tablespoons avocado oil
- 2 garlic cloves, minced
- A pinch of salt and black pepper
- 6 eggs, whisked
- ¼ cup heavy cream
- 1 cup cheddar cheese, grated
- 1 green onion, chopped

Directions:

Set the instant pot on Sauté mode, add the oil, heat it up, add the garlic and the broccoli, stir and sauté for 4 minutes. In a bowl, mix the eggs with the cream, salt and pepper, whisk well and pour over the broccoli mix in the pot. Put the lid on and cook on High for 35 minutes. Release the pressure naturally for 10 minutes, sprinkle the cheese and the onion all over, leave aside for a few minutes more, divide between plates and serve.

Nutrition: calories 247, fat 19, fiber 0.5, carbs 2.3, protein 15

Bell Peppers and Cauliflower Salad

Preparation time: 10 minutes | Cooking time: 20 minutes | Servings: 4

Ingredients:

- 1 cauliflower head, florets separated
- 1 tablespoon avocado oil
- 2 spring onions, chopped
- ¼ red bell pepper, sliced
- ¼ yellow bell pepper, sliced
- ¼ green bell pepper, sliced
- A pinch of salt and black pepper
- 2 eggs

Directions:

Set the instant pot on Sauté mode, add the oil, heat it up, add the bell peppers and sauté them for 4 minutes. Add the rest of the ingredients, toss a bit, put the lid on and cook on High for 15 minutes. Release the pressure naturally for 10 minutes, divide the mix into bowls and serve for breakfast.

Nutrition: calories 63, fat 3, fiber 2.3, carbs 6, protein 4.5

Cauliflower Hash

Preparation time: 10 minutes | Cooking time: 15 minutes | Servings: 4

Ingredients:

- A pinch of salt and black pepper
- 2 cups cauliflower, riced
- 1 teaspoon red bell pepper, chopped
- 1 teaspoon green bell pepper, chopped
- ½ tablespoon olive oil
- 1 cup black olives, pitted and chopped
- 1 cup cheddar cheese, shredded

Directions:

Set your instant pot on sauté mode, add the oil, heat it up, add the cauliflower rice and cook it for 2-3 minutes. Add the rest of the ingredients except the cheese, toss a bit, put the lid on and cook on High for 12 minutes. Release the pressure naturally for 10 minutes, divide the hash between plates and serve.

Nutrition: calories 199, fat 14.9, fiber 3, carbs 7.6, protein 8.9

Scallions and Broccoli Mix

Preparation time: 10 minutes | Cooking time: 20 minutes | Servings: 4

Ingredients:

- 1 pound broccoli florets, roughly chopped
- 4 eggs, whisked
- 1 tablespoon sweet paprika
- 1 tablespoon avocado oil
- 2 scallions, chopped
- 1 cup cheddar cheese, shredded

Directions:

Set the instant pot on Sauté mode, add the oil, heat it up, add the scallions and the broccoli, toss, and sauté for 5 minutes. Add the eggs and the paprika, toss, put the lid on and cook on High for 15 minutes more. Release the pressure naturally for 10 minutes, sprinkle the cheese on top, leave the mix aside for a couple more minutes, divide it between plates and serve for breakfast.

Nutrition: calories 227, fat 14.8, fiber 4, carbs 6.7, protein 16

Pork Hash

Preparation time: 10 minutes | Cooking time: 20 minutes | Servings: 4

Ingredients:

- 2 tablespoons olive oil
- 1 spring onion, chopped
- 2 garlic cloves, minced
- 1 pound pork meat, ground
- 1 red bell pepper, chopped
- 1 green bell pepper, chopped
- ½ teaspoon Italian seasoning
- 2 tablespoons veggie stock
- 1 tablespoon cilantro, chopped

Directions:

Set your instant pot on sauté mode, add the oil, heat it up, add the onion and the garlic and sauté for 2 minutes. Add the meat and brown it for 3 minutes more. Add the rest of the ingredients, put the lid on and cook on High for 15 minutes more. Release the pressure naturally for 10 minutes, divide the hash between plates and serve for breakfast.

Nutrition: calories 104, fat 7.4, fiber 0.9, carbs 5.4, protein 1

Creamy Eggs Ramekins

Preparation time: 10 minutes | Cooking time: 5 minutes | Servings: 4

Ingredients:

- 2 tablespoons ghee, melted
- ¼ cup cream cheese
- 2 tablespoons heavy cream
- 4 eggs, whisked
- 1 teaspoon hot paprika
- 1 tablespoon chives, chopped
- A pinch of salt and black pepper
- 1 cup water

Directions:

In a bowl, combine the cream cheese with the eggs and the rest of the ingredients except the chives and the water and whisk well. Divide this into 4 ramekins and sprinkle the chives on top. Put the water in the instant pot, add the steamer basket inside, put the ramekins in the pot, put the lid on and cook on High for 5 minutes. Release the pressure naturally for 10 minutes and serve the eggs hot.

Nutrition: calories 196, fat 18.6, fiber 0, carbs 1, protein 6.8

Avocado and Broccoli Salad

Preparation time: 10 minutes | Cooking time: 16 minutes | Servings: 4

Ingredients:

- 2 cup broccoli florets
- ¼ cup coconut milk
- ½ cup cheddar cheese, shredded
- A pinch of salt and black pepper
- 1 tablespoon chives, chopped
- 1 tablespoon avocado oil
- 1 tablespoon balsamic vinegar
- 1 avocado, peeled, pitted and cubed
- 1 cup baby arugula

Directions:

In your instant pot, combine the broccoli with the except the milk, cheese, salt and pepper, toss, put the lid on and cook on High for 12 minutes. Release the pressure naturally for 10 minutes, cool the broccoli mix a bit, transfer it to a bowl, add the avocado and the remaining ingredients, toss and serve.

Nutrition: calories 216, fat 18.7, fiber 5, carbs 7.6, protein 7

Coconut Blueberry Pudding

Preparation time: 10 minutes | Cooking time: 25 minutes | Servings: 4

Ingredients:

- 1 and ½ cups coconut flour
- Zest of 1 lime, grated
- 2 teaspoons baking powder
- ½ cup ghee, melted
- ¾ cup swerve
- 1 teaspoon vanilla extract
- 1 egg, whisked
- ½ cup coconut milk
- 2 cups blueberries
- 1 cup water

Directions:

In a bowl, mix all the ingredients except the water, whisk well and divide into 4 ramekins. Add the water to your instant pot, add the steamer basket, add the ramekins inside, put the lid on and cook on High for 25 minutes. Release the pressure naturally for 10 minutes, and serve the puddings for breakfast.

Nutrition: calories 356, fat 34, fiber 2.5, carbs 10, protein 2.7

Bacon and Eggs

Preparation time: 10 minutes | Cooking time: 15 minutes | Servings: 4

Ingredients:

- 1 shallot, chopped
- 1 and ½ cups bacon, chopped
- 2 cups cheddar cheese, shredded
- 4 eggs, whisked
- 1 cup almond milk
- 1 tablespoon avocado oil
- A pinch of salt and black pepper

Directions:

Set the instant pot on Sauté mode, add the oil, heat it up, add the bacon and the shallot and cook for 2-3 minutes. Add the rest of the ingredients, toss, put the lid on and cook on High for 12 minutes. Release the pressure naturally for 10 minutes, divide the mix between plates and serve.

Nutrition: calories 392, fat 37, fiber 1.4, carbs 4.6, protein 21

Broccoli and Cheese Pancake

Preparation time: 10 minutes | *Cooking time:* 25 minutes | *Servings:* 4

Ingredients:

- 2 cups coconut flour
- A pinch of salt and black pepper
- 3 eggs, whisked
- 1 teaspoon baking soda
- 1 and ½ cups almond milk
- 1 cup mozzarella, shredded
- 1 cup broccoli florets, grated
- Cooking spray

Directions:

In a bowl, mix the eggs with the eggs and the rest of the ingredients except the cooking spray and whisk well. Grease the instant pot with the cooking spray, add the pancake mix, spread, put the lid on and cook on High for 25 minutes. Release the pressure naturally for 10 minutes, divide the pancake between plates and serve for breakfast.

Nutrition: calories 76, fat 4.8, fiber 0.6, carbs 2, protein 6.8

Tomato and Peppers Salad

Preparation time: 10 minutes | *Cooking time:* 10 minutes | *Servings:* 4

Ingredients:

- A pinch of salt and black pepper
- 3 cups baby spinach, chopped
- 1 pound cherry tomatoes, cubed
- 3 green onions, chopped
- 1 tablespoon olive oil
- 1 tablespoon balsamic vinegar
- ½ pound mixed bell peppers, cut into strips

Directions:

Set the instant pot on Sauté mode, add the oil, heat it up, add the onions and sauté for 2 minutes. Add the tomatoes and the rest of the ingredients, put the lid on and cook on High for 8 minutes. Release the pressure naturally for 10 minutes, divide the mix into bowls and serve for breakfast.

Nutrition: calories 60, fat 8.1, fiber 2, carbs 6.1, protein 1.9

Chili Frittata

Preparation time: 10 minutes | Cooking time: 30 minutes | Servings: 4

Ingredients:

- 1 cup heavy cream
- 4 eggs, whisked
- 10 ounces canned green chilies
- A pinch of salt and black pepper
- ½ teaspoon sweet paprika
- 1 teaspoon chili powder
- 1 tablespoon cilantro, chopped
- 1 tablespoon avocado oil

Directions:

In a bowl, mix the eggs with the rest of the ingredients except the oil and whisk well. Grease the instant pot with the oil, pour the eggs mixture, spread, put the lid on and cook on High for 30 minutes. Release the pressure naturally for 10 minutes, divide the frittata between plates and serve for breakfast.

Nutrition: calories 404, fat 20.2, fiber 8.9, carbs 11.1, protein 14.6

Cheesy Beef Casserole

Preparation time: 10 minutes | Cooking time: 25 minutes | Servings: 6

Ingredients:

- 1 pound beef, ground
- 4 eggs, whisked
- 1 red bell pepper, chopped
- ½ cup green onions, chopped
- 1 tablespoon olive oil
- 1 cup mozzarella cheese, shredded
- 1 tablespoon cilantro, chopped

Directions:

Set your instant pot on sauté mode, add the oil, heat it up, add the meat and brown for 5 minutes. Add the rest of the ingredients except the cheese and the cilantro and toss. Sprinkle the cheese on top, put the lid on and cook on High for 20 minutes. Release the pressure naturally for 10 minutes, divide the mix between plates, sprinkle the cilantro on top and serve.

Nutrition: calories 224, fat 10.9, fiber 0.5, carbs 2.5, protein 28.2

Asparagus and Eggs Mix

Preparation time: 5 minutes | Cooking time: 20 minutes | Servings: 6

Ingredients:

- 1 asparagus stalk, halved
- 6 eggs, whisked
- ¼ cup scallions, chopped
- 1 red chili pepper, chopped
- A pinch of salt and black pepper
- ¼ teaspoon chili powder
- 1 tablespoon olive oil

Directions:

Set the instant pot on Sauté mode, add the oil, heat it up, add the asparagus and the scallions and cook for 2-3 minutes. Add the eggs and the rest of the ingredients, toss, put the lid on and cook on High for 15 minutes. Release the pressure fast for 5 minutes, divide the mix between plates and serve.

Nutrition: calories 85, fat 6.7, fiber 0.2, carbs 0.8, protein 5.6

Chia and Blueberries Bowls

Preparation time: 5 minutes | Cooking time: 10 minutes | Servings: 4

Ingredients:

- ¼ cup chia seeds
- 1 cup blueberries
- 1/3 cup almonds, chopped
- 1 and ½ cup almond milk
- 1 teaspoon vanilla extract
- 2 tablespoons stevia

Directions:

In your instant pot, combine the chia seeds with the rest of the ingredients, put the lid on and cook on High for 10 minutes. Release the pressure fast for 5 minutes, divide the mix into bowls and serve for breakfast.

Nutrition: calories 70, fat 4.1, fiber 1.9, carbs 4.3, protein 2

Almond Cocoa and Strawberries Mix

Preparation time: 10 minutes | Cooking time: 10 minutes | Servings: 4

Ingredients:

- 3 cups almond milk
- ½ cup coconut cream
- 2 and ½ tablespoon cocoa powder
- 2 cups strawberries, halved
- 1 teaspoon vanilla extract
- 1 teaspoon cinnamon powder

Directions:

In your instant pot, combine the almond milk with the rest of the ingredients, toss, put the lid on and cook on High for 10 minutes. Release the pressure naturally for 10 minutes, divide the strawberry mix into bowls and serve for breakfast.

Nutrition: calories 312, fat 14.5, fiber 4.6, carbs 7.9, protein 5.6

Coconut Yogurt Mix

Preparation time: 5 minutes | Cooking time: 5 minutes | Servings: 2

Ingredients:

- 1 cup coconut milk
- ½ cup coconut, unsweetened and flaked
- 1 cup yogurt
- ½ teaspoon stevia
- ¼ teaspoon vanilla extract
- ½ teaspoon cinnamon powder

Directions:

In your instant pot, combine the coconut milk with the coconut and the rest of the ingredients, toss, put the lid on and cook on High for 5 minutes. Release the pressure fast for 5 minutes, divide the yogurt mix into bowls and serve.

Nutrition: calories 218, fat 18.4, fiber 2.2, carbs 6.7, protein 5.2

Artichokes Pudding

Preparation time: 10 minutes | Cooking time: 15 minutes | Servings: 4

Ingredients:

- 2 cups almond milk
- ¼ cup coconut cream
- 1 and ½ cups canned artichokes, drained and chopped
- 1 teaspoon sweet paprika
- A pinch of salt and black pepper
- 1 tablespoon chives, chopped

Directions:

In your instant pot, mix the almond milk with cream and the rest of the ingredients, put the lid on and cook on High for 15 minutes. Release the pressure naturally for 10 minutes, divide the mix between plates and serve.

Nutrition: calories 312, fat 23.4, fiber 3.2, carbs 7.3, protein 3.2

Scotch Eggs and Tomato Passata

Preparation time: 6 minutes | Cooking time: 18 minutes | Servings: 4

Ingredients:

- 1 pound pork, ground
- A pinch of salt and black pepper
- 1 teaspoon cilantro, chopped
- 1 teaspoon hot paprika
- 4 eggs, hard boiled and peeled
- 1 tablespoon avocado oil
- 1 cup tomato passata

Directions:

In a bowl, mix the pork with the rest of the ingredients except the eggs, tomato passata and the oil and stir well. Divide the mix into 4 balls and flatten them on a working surface. Divide the eggs on each pork ball and wrap them well. Set the instant pot on Sauté mode, add the oil, heat it up, add the scotch eggs and brown them for 2 minutes on each side. Add the tomato passata, put the lid on and cook on High for 12 minutes. Release pressure fast for 6 minutes, divide the mix between plates and serve for breakfast.

Nutrition: calories 245, fat 8.9, fiber 1.1, carbs 3.9, protein 36

Parsley Cauliflower Mix

Preparation time: 10 *minutes* | *Cooking time:* 20 *minutes* | *Servings:* 4

Ingredients:

- 2 cups cauliflower florets
- 2 ounces cheddar cheese, shredded
- 1 teaspoon garlic powder
- 1 teaspoon chili powder
- 2 eggs, whisked
- 1 tablespoon parsley, chopped
- 1 tablespoon avocado oil
- ½ cup heavy cream
- A pinch of salt and black pepper

Directions:

Set your instant pot on sauté mode, add the oil, heat it up, add the cauliflower, garlic and chili powder and cook for 5 minutes. Add the rest of the ingredients, toss, put the lid on and cook on High for 15 minutes. Release the pressure naturally for 10 minutes, divide the mix into bowls and serve for breakfast.

Nutrition: calories 164, fat 13.1, fiber 1.7, carbs 4.6, protein 7.9

Pork Pie

Preparation time: 10 *minutes* | *Cooking time:* 30 *minutes* | *Servings:* 4

Ingredients:

- ½ cup heavy cream
- A pinch of salt and black pepper
- 4 eggs, whisked
- 2 cups pork meat, ground and browned
- 2 green onions, chopped
- 1 cup cheddar cheese, shredded
- 1 cup water

Directions:

In a bowl, mix the eggs with the rest of the ingredients except the water, whisk well and spread into a pie pan. Add the water to your instant pot, add the trivet, add the pan inside, put the lid on and cook on High for 30 minutes. Release the pressure naturally for 10 minutes, divide the mix between plates and serve hot for breakfast.

Nutrition: calories 231, fat 19.3, fiber 0.2, carbs 1.7, protein 13

Ginger Cauliflower Rice Pudding

Preparation time: 10 minutes | Cooking time: 15 minutes | Servings: 4

Ingredients:

- 2 cups almond milk
- 1 cup cauliflower rice
- 1 teaspoon cinnamon powder
- 1 tablespoon ginger, grated
- 3 tablespoons stevia
- 1 teaspoon vanilla extract

Directions:

In your instant pot, mix the cauliflower rice with the milk and the other ingredients, toss, put the lid on and cook on High for 15 minutes. Release the pressure naturally for 10 minutes, stir the pudding, divide it into bowls and serve.

Nutrition: calories 284, fat 28.7, fiber 2.8, carbs 7.7, protein 2.9

Bok Choy Bowls

Preparation time: 10 minutes | Cooking time: 20 minutes | Servings: 4

Ingredients:

- 1 and ½ cups veggie stock
- 2 cups bok choy, roughly torn
- 2 tablespoons ginger, grated
- 2 garlic cloves, minced
- 1 tablespoon coconut aminos
- 1 tablespoon sweet paprika
- 2 tomatoes, cubed
- A pinch of salt and black pepper

Directions:

In your instant pot, mix the bok choy with the stock and the rest of the ingredients, toss, put the lid on and cook on High for 20 minutes. Release the pressure naturally for 10 minutes, divide the mix into bowls and serve for breakfast.

Nutrition: calories 89, fat 6.8, fiber 2.1, carbs 6.1, protein 1.7

Mushroom and Avocado Salad
Preparation time: 10 minutes | Cooking time: 20 minutes | Servings: 4

Ingredients:

- 2 avocados, pitted, peeled and cubed
- 1 tablespoon olive oil
- 1 tablespoon chives, chopped
- A pinch of salt and black pepper
- ½ pound white mushrooms, sliced
- 1 tablespoon balsamic vinegar
- ½ cup veggie stock
- 1 cup baby arugula

Directions:

Set the instant pot on Sauté mode, add the oil, heat it up, add the mushrooms and cook for 4 minutes. Add the rest of the ingredients except the avocado and the arugula, put the lid on and cook on High for 15 minutes. Release the pressure naturally for 10 minutes, transfer the mix to a bowl, add the avocado and the arugula, toss and serve for breakfast.

Nutrition: calories 250, fat 23.3, fiber 6.4, carbs 7.6, protein 3.8

Salmon and Eggs Mix
Preparation time: 10 minutes | Cooking time: 12 minutes | Servings: 4

Ingredients:

- 4 ounces smoked salmon, skinless, boneless and cut into strips
- 4 eggs
- A pinch of salt and black pepper
- ½ cup coconut cream
- 1 tablespoon chives, chopped
- 1 tablespoon cilantro, chopped
- Cooking spray

Directions:

In a bowl, mix the salmon with the eggs and the rest of the ingredients except the cooking spray and whisk well. Grease the instant pot with the cooking spray, pour the salmon mix, spread, put the lid on and cook on High for 12 minutes. Release the pressure naturally for 10 minutes, divide the mix between plates and serve.

Nutrition: calories 167, fat 12.9, fiber 0.7, carbs 2.1, protein 11.4

Italian Beef and Green Beans Mix

Preparation time: 10 minutes | Cooking time: 30 minutes | Servings: 6

Ingredients:

- 2 spring onions chopped
- 1 red bell pepper, chopped
- 1 pound beef, ground
- ½ cup veggie stock
- A pinch of salt and black pepper
- 1 tablespoon Italian seasoning
- 1 tablespoon cilantro, chopped
- 1 teaspoon olive oil
- ½ pound green beans, trimmed and halved

Directions:

Set your instant pot on sauté mode, add the oil, heat it up, add the meat, Italian seasoning, salt and pepper and brown for 5 minutes. Add the rest of the ingredients, toss, put the lid on and cook on High for 25 minutes. Release the pressure naturally for 10 minutes, divide everything between plates and serve for breakfast.

Nutrition: calories 259, fat 9.4, fiber 2.4, carbs 6.7, protein 35.8

Herbed Mushroom Mix

Preparation time: 10 minutes | Cooking time: 20 minutes | Servings: 4

Ingredients:

- 1 and ½ pounds brown mushrooms, chopped
- 2 tablespoons chicken stock
- A pinch of salt and black pepper
- 1 tablespoon olive oil
- ½ teaspoon garlic powder
- ½ teaspoon basil, dried
- 1 teaspoon rosemary, chopped
- 1 red bell pepper, cut into strips

Directions:

Set your instant pot on sauté mode, add the oil, heat it up, add the mushrooms, stir and sauté for 5 minutes. Add the rest of the ingredients, put the lid on and cook on High for 15 minutes. Release the pressure naturally for 10 minutes, divide the mix between plates and serve for breakfast.

Nutrition: calories 42, fat 3.7, fiber 0.6, carbs 2.7, protein 0.4

Creamy Zucchini Pan

Preparation time: 10 minutes | Cooking time: 20 minutes | Servings: 4

Ingredients:

- 4 zucchinis, sliced
- 1 tablespoon avocado oil
- 1 shallot, minced
- ¼ cup heavy cream
- 2 tablespoons parsley, chopped
- 6 eggs, whisked
- 2 tablespoons cheddar, grated
- A pinch of salt and black pepper

Directions:

Set the instant pot on Sauté mode, add the oil, heat it up, add the shallot and sauté for 2-3 minutes. Add the zucchinis and the rest of the ingredients, toss, put the lid on and cook on High for 15 minutes. Release the pressure naturally for 10 minutes, divide the mix between plates and serve for breakfast.

Nutrition: calories 163, fat 10.4, fiber 2.4, carbs 7.7, protein 11.8

Leeks and Pork Mix

Preparation time: 10 minutes | Cooking time: 30 minutes | Servings: 4

Ingredients:

- 1 pound pork meat, ground
- ¼ cup coconut cream
- 2 leeks, chopped
- 4 eggs, whisked
- 1 tablespoon sweet paprika
- 1 tablespoon chives, chopped
- A pinch of salt and black pepper
- ¼ teaspoon garlic powder
- 1 tablespoon olive oil

Directions:

Set your instant pot on sauté mode, add the oil, heat it up, add the leeks and sauté for 5 minutes. Add the meat and brown for 4-5 minutes more. Add the eggs and the rest of the ingredients, toss, put the lid on and cook on High for 20 minutes. Release the pressure naturally for 10 minutes, divide the mix between plates and serve for breakfast.

Nutrition: calories 160, fat 11.8, fiber 1.8, carbs 7.1, protein 6.9

Cardamom Walnuts Pudding

Preparation time: 5 minutes | Cooking time: 10 minutes | Servings: 2

Ingredients:

- 1 teaspoon cardamom, ground
- ½ cup walnuts, chopped
- 1 teaspoon swerve
- 1 and ½ cups coconut cream
- 2 tablespoons almond meal

Directions:

In your instant pot, mix the cream with the cardamom and the rest of the ingredients, toss, put the lid on and cook on High for 10 minutes. Release the pressure fast for 5 minutes, divide everything into bowls and serve.

Nutrition: calories 231, fat 21.9, fiber 3.2, carbs 5.1, protein 8.9

Basil Eggs Mix

Preparation time: 5 minutes | Cooking time: 15 minutes | Servings: 4

Ingredients:

- 2 tablespoons basil, chopped
- Cooking spray
- A pinch of salt and black pepper
- 4 eggs, whisked
- 1 cup cheddar cheese, shredded
- 1 teaspoon chili powder

Directions:

Grease the instant pot with the cooking spray, add the eggs and the rest of the ingredients, toss, put the lid on and cook on High for 15 minutes. Release the pressure fast for 5 minutes, divide the mix between plates and serve for breakfast.

Nutrition: calories 180, fat 14, fiber 0.3, carbs 1.1, protein 12.7

Creamy Blueberries and Nuts

Preparation time: 5 minutes | Cooking time: 8 minutes | Servings: 6

Ingredients:

- ½ cup walnuts, chopped
- ½ cups almonds, chopped
- 2 teaspoons swerve
- 1 cup blueberries
- 1 teaspoon vanilla extract
- 1 cup coconut cream

Directions:

In your instant pot, combine the walnuts with the almonds and the rest of the ingredients, toss, put the lid on and cook on High for 8 minutes. Release the pressure fast for 5 minutes, divide the mix into bowls and serve for breakfast.

Nutrition: calories 218, fat 19.7, fiber 3.2, carbs 5.8, protein 5.3

Kale and Bok Choy Muffins

Preparation time: 10 minutes | Cooking time: 20 minutes | Servings: 4

Ingredients:

- ½ cup almond milk
- 4 eggs, whisked
- 1 tablespoon avocado oil
- A pinch of salt and black pepper
- ½ cup bok choy, chopped
- ½ cup kale, chopped
- 1 tablespoon chives, chopped
- 1 and ½ cups water

Directions:

In a bowl, mix the almond milk with the eggs and the rest of the ingredients except the water and the oil and stir well. Grease a muffin tray with the oil and pour the muffin mix inside. Add the water to your instant pot, add the trivet, add muffin tray inside, put the lid on and cook on High for 20 minutes. Release the pressure naturally for 10 minutes, cool the muffins down and serve for breakfast.

Nutrition: calories 142, fat 12, fiber 1.1, carbs 3.3, protein 6.7

Spinach and Artichokes Muffins

Preparation time: 10 minutes | Cooking time: 20 minutes | Servings: 12

Ingredients:

- 1 cup baby spinach, chopped
- 1 cup canned artichoke hearts, drained and chopped
- A pinch of salt and black pepper
- 1 and ½ cups water
- Cooking spray
- 3 cups almond flour
- 1 teaspoon baking soda
- 4 eggs

Directions:

In a bowl, mix the spinach with the artichokes and the rest of the ingredients except the water and the cooking spray and stir well. Grease a muffin tray with the cooking spray and pour the muffin mix inside. Add the water to your instant pot, add the trivet, add the muffin tray inside, put the lid on and cook on High for 20 minutes. Release the pressure naturally for 10 minutes, cool the muffins down and serve for breakfast.

Nutrition: calories 66, fat 4.5, fiber 0.2, carbs 0.6, protein 5.8

Mozzarella and Kale Muffins

Preparation time: 10 minutes | Cooking time: 20 minutes | Servings: 4

Ingredients:

- Cooking spray
- 2 cups water
- 1 cup mozzarella cheese, grated
- 4 eggs, whisked
- ½ teaspoon basil, dried
- ¼ teaspoon baking soda
- 1 cup almond flour
- ¼ cup kale, chopped
- A pinch of salt and black pepper
- ½ cup almond milk

Directions:

In a bowl, mix the mozzarella with the eggs and the rest of the ingredients except the water and the cooking spray and whisk well. Grease a muffin tray with the cooking spray and pour the muffins mix inside. Add the water to your instant pot, add the trivet, add the muffin tray inside, put the lid on and cook on High for 20 minutes. Release the pressure naturally for 10 minutes, divide the muffins between plates and serve for breakfast.

Nutrition: calories 155, fat 12.9, fiber 0.7, carbs 2.7, protein 8.4

Chicken Bowls

Preparation time: 10 minutes | Cooking time: 15 minutes | Servings: 4

Ingredients:

- 1 avocado, peeled and cut into wedges
- 2 tomatoes, cubed
- 1 and ½ cups baby spinach
- A pinch of salt and black pepper
- 2 chicken breasts, skinless, boneless and cubed
- 2 tablespoons olive oil
- 2 tablespoons chicken stock
- ¼ cup tomato passata
- 1 shallot, chopped

Directions:

Set your instant pot on sauté mode, add the oil, heat it up, add the shallot and sauté for 2 minutes. Add the chicken, stock and tomato passata, put the lid on and cook on High for 13 minutes. Release the pressure naturally for 10 minutes, transfer the chicken mix to a bowl, add the remaining ingredients, toss and serve for breakfast.

Nutrition: calories 1, fa78t 17, fiber 4.6, carbs 7.6, protein 1.7

Coconut Pudding

Preparation time: 5 minutes | Cooking time: 5 minutes | Servings: 6

Ingredients:

- 2 cups coconut milk
- 1 cup coconut cream
- ¼ cup walnuts, chopped
- ½ cup coconut, unsweetened and shredded
- 4 teaspoons swerve

Directions:

In your instant pot, combine the coconut milk with the rest of the ingredients, toss, put the lid on and cook on High for 5 minutes. Release the pressure fast for 5 minutes, divide the pudding into bowls and serve.

Nutrition: calories 332, fat 33.8, fiber 3.6, carbs 7.8, protein 4.2

Zucchini Spread

Preparation time: 10 minutes | Cooking time: 12 minutes | Servings: 4

Ingredients:

- 4 zucchinis, sliced
- A pinch of salt and black pepper
- ½ cup heavy cream
- ½ cup cream cheese, soft
- 2 garlic cloves, minced
- ½ cup veggie stock
- 1 tablespoon avocado oil
- 1 tablespoon dill, chopped

Directions:

In your instant pot, mix the zucchinis with the stock, salt and pepper, put the lid on and cook on High for 12 minutes. Release the pressure naturally for 10 minutes, drain the zucchinis, transfer them to a blender, add the rest of the ingredients, pulse, divide into bowls and serve as a morning spread.

Nutrition: calories 193, fat 16.5, fiber 2.5, carbs 7.8, protein 5.2

Tomato And Zucchini Salad

Preparation time: 10 minutes | Cooking time: 10 minutes | Servings: 4

Ingredients:

- 2 spring onions, chopped
- 1 pound cherry tomatoes, roughly cubed
- 2 zucchinis, sliced
- 1 tablespoon olive oil
- 2 garlic cloves, minced
- 1 tablespoon rosemary, chopped
- 1 tablespoon basil, chopped
- ½ cup tomato passata
- 1 tablespoon chives, chopped
- A pinch of sea salt and black pepper

Directions:

Set your instant pot on sauté mode add the oil, heat it up, add the spring onions and the garlic and sauté for 2-3 minutes. Add tomatoes, zucchinis and the rest of the ingredients except the chives, put the lid on and cook on High for 8 minutes. Release the pressure naturally for 10 minutes, divide the mix into bowls and serve for breakfast with the chives sprinkled on top.

Nutrition: calories 86, fat 4.1, fiber 3.6, carbs 5.8, protein 3

Turkey Bowls

Preparation time: 10 minutes | Cooking time: 20 minutes | Servings: 2

Ingredients:

- 1 tablespoon olive oil
- 2 cups okra, sliced
- ½ cup chicken stock
- 2 cups yellow bell pepper, chopped
- A pinch of salt and black pepper
- 1 turkey breast, skinless, boneless and cubed
- 2 tablespoons oregano, chopped
- 1 tablespoon thyme, chopped
- ½ cup balsamic vinegar

Directions:

Set the instant pot on sauté mode, add the oil, heat it up, add the turkey and brown for 5 minutes. Add the okra and the rest of the ingredients, put the lid on and cook on High for 15 minutes. Release the pressure naturally for 10 minutes, divide the mix into bowls and serve for breakfast.

Nutrition: calories 171, fat 8.2, fiber 2.6, carbs 7.8, protein 3.9

Cheesy Tomato and Radish Salad

Preparation time: 10 minutes | Cooking time: 10 minutes | Servings: 4

Ingredients:

- ¼ cup radishes, sliced
- 1 pound cherry tomatoes, halved
- 1 tablespoon basil, chopped
- 1 tablespoon olive oil
- 1 tablespoon chives, chopped
- ½ cup mozzarella, shredded
- A pinch of salt and black pepper

Directions:

In your instant pot, mix the radishes with the tomatoes and the rest of the ingredients except the mozzarella and toss. Sprinkle the cheese on top, put the lid on and cook on High for 10 minutes. Release the pressure naturally for 10 minutes, divide the salad into bowls and serve for breakfast.

Nutrition: calories 62, fat 4.4, fiber 1.5, carbs 4.9, protein 2.1

Pork and Kale Hash

Preparation time: 10 minutes | Cooking time: 15 minutes | Servings: 4

Ingredients:

- 1 tablespoon avocado oil
- 1 spring onion, chopped
- 2 cups pork meat, ground
- 2 garlic cloves, minced
- ½ cup beef stock
- A pinch of salt and black pepper
- 1 pound kale, torn

Directions:

Set your instant pot on sauté mode, add the oil, heat it up, add the onion, garlic and the meat and brown for 5 minutes. Add the rest of the ingredients, toss, put the lid on and cook on High for 10 minutes. Release the pressure naturally for 10 minutes, divide the mix between plates and serve.

Nutrition: calories 66, fat 5.3, fiber 2, carbs 6.5, protein 3.8

Sweet Zucchini Mix

Preparation time: 10 minutes | Cooking time: 10 minutes | Servings: 4

Ingredients:

- 1 and ½ cups coconut cream
- 1 teaspoon nutmeg, ground
- 4 zucchinis, sliced
- 2 tablespoons swerve
- ¼ cup walnuts, chopped

Directions:

In your instant pot, combine the cream with the zucchinis and the rest of the ingredients, put the lid on and cook on High for 10 minutes. Release the pressure naturally for 10 minutes, divide the mix into bowls and serve.

Nutrition: calories 83, fat 8.2, fiber 2.8, carbs 7.6, protein 4.3

Turkey Omelet

Preparation time: 10 minutes | Cooking time: 15 minutes | Servings: 4

Ingredients:

- 1 cup turkey breast, skinless, boneless and cut into strips
- 1 tomato, chopped
- 2 bacon slices, cooked and crumbled
- 4 eggs, whisked
- 1 small avocado, pitted, peeled and chopped
- A pinch of salt and black pepper
- 2 tablespoons olive oil

Directions:

Set your instant pot on sauté mode, add half of the oil, heat it up, add the meat and cook for 5 minutes. Add the rest of the ingredients, toss, spread the mix into the pot, put the lid on and cook on High for 10 minutes. Release the pressure naturally for 10 minutes, divide the omelet between plates and serve.

Nutrition: calories 228, fat 21.2, fiber 3.6, carbs 5.3, protein 6.6

Strawberries and Nuts Salad

Preparation time: 10 minutes | Cooking time: 10 minutes | Servings: 4

Ingredients:

- ½ cup almonds, chopped
- ½ cup walnuts, chopped
- 2 cups strawberries, halved
- 1 tablespoon stevia
- ½ teaspoon nutmeg, ground
- 1 cup coconut cream

Directions:

In your instant pot, mix the strawberries with the cream and the rest of the ingredients, put the lid on and cook on Low for 10 minutes. Release the pressure naturally for 10 minutes, divide the mix into bowls and serve.

Nutrition: calories 328, fat 29.8, fiber 5.4, carbs 7.6, protein 8.1

Eggs, Leeks and Turkey Mix

Preparation time: 10 minutes | Cooking time: 15 minutes | Servings: 4

Ingredients:

- 2 leeks, chopped
- ½ cup chicken stock
- 2 tablespoons olive oil
- 2 garlic cloves, minced
- 8 eggs, whisked
- 1 turkey breast, skinless, boneless and cut into strips

Directions:

Set your instant pot on Sauté mode, add the oil, heat it up, add the leeks, garlic and the meat and brown for 5 minutes. Add the rest of the ingredients, toss, put the lid on and cook on High for 10 minutes. Release the pressure naturally for 10 minutes, divide the mix between plates and serve.

Nutrition: calories 216, fat 16, fiber 0.8, carbs 7.6, protein 11.9

Sweet Berries Bowls

Preparation time: 10 minutes | Cooking time: 12 minutes | Servings: 6

Ingredients:

- 3 tablespoons coconut flakes, unsweetened
- 1 cup strawberries
- 1 cup blackberries
- 2 cups almond milk
- 1 teaspoon vanilla extract
- 1 teaspoon swerve

Directions:

In your instant pot, mix the berries with the coconut and the rest of the ingredients, put the lid on and cook on Low for 12 minutes. Release the pressure naturally for 10 minutes, divide the mix into bowls and serve.

Nutrition: calories 213, fat 20.1, fiber 3.7, carbs 6.7, protein 2.4

Mushroom and Okra Omelet

Preparation time: 10 minutes | Cooking time: 15 minutes | Servings: 2

Ingredients:

- 1 pound white mushrooms, sliced
- 2 spring onions, chopped
- 2 garlic cloves, minced
- 1 tablespoon avocado oil
- 2 chili peppers, minced
- 1 cup okra
- ½ cup cilantro, chopped
- 4 eggs, whisked

Directions:

Set your instant pot on sauté mode, add the oil, heat it up, add the onions and garlic and sauté for 2 minutes. Add the mushrooms and sauté for 2 minutes more. Add the rest of the ingredients, toss, spread the mix into the instant pot, put the lid on and cook on High for 10 minutes. Release the pressure naturally for 10 minutes, divide the omelet between plates and serve.

Nutrition: calories 108, fat 5.2, fiber 2.4, carbs 4.7, protein 9.9

Cocoa Oatmeal

Preparation time: 10 minutes | Cooking time: 10 minutes | Servings: 6

Ingredients:

- 1 cup almond milk
- 1 cup coconut cream
- 1 cup coconut flakes, unsweetened
- 2 tablespoons stevia
- 1 teaspoon cocoa powder
- 2 teaspoons vanilla extract

Directions:

In your instant pot, mix the almond milk with the rest of the ingredients, put the lid on and cook on High for 10 minutes. Release the pressure naturally for 10 minutes, divide the mix into bowls and serve.

Nutrition: calories 236, fat 23.6, fiber 3.1, carbs 6.5, protein 2.3

Coconut Oatmeal

Preparation time: 5 minutes | Cooking time: 10 minutes | Servings: 6

Ingredients:

- 1 cup coconut, unsweetened and shredded
- 1 cup coconut milk
- 1 cup walnuts, chopped
- ½ cup almonds, chopped
- 1 cup coconut cream
- Seeds from 1 pomegranate

Directions:

In your instant pot, mix the coconut with the milk and the rest of the ingredients, toss, put the lid on and cook on High for 10 minutes. Release the pressure fast for 5 minutes, divide the mix into bowls and serve for breakfast.

Nutrition: calories 406, fat 30.2, fiber 5.4, carbs 6.8, protein 9

Broccoli and Almonds Mix

Preparation time: 5 minutes | Cooking time: 15 minutes | Servings: 4

Ingredients:

- 1 cup broccoli florets
- ½ cup coconut flakes
- 1 cup heavy cream
- ½ cup almonds, toasted and chopped
- 2 eggs, whisked
- Cooking spray

Directions:

Grease the instant pot with the cooking spray, add the broccoli and almonds and the pour the eggs mixed with the heavy cream on top. Sprinkle the coconut on top, put the lid on and cook on High for 15 minutes. Release the pressure fast for 5 minutes, divide the mix between plates and serve.

Nutrition: calories 248, fat 22.8, fiber 3, carbs 6.6, protein 6.9

Mushroom and Cauliflower Rice Salad

Preparation time: 10 minutes | Cooking time: 20 minutes | Servings: 4

Ingredients:

- 2 shallots, chopped
- 2 tablespoons avocado oil
- 2 cups white mushrooms, sliced
- 2 tablespoons lemon juice
- A pinch of salt and black pepper
- 4 garlic cloves, minced
- 1 cup cauliflower rice
- 1 cup veggie stock
- 1 tablespoon chives, chopped

Directions:

Set your instant pot on sauté mode, add the oil, heat it up, add the shallots, garlic and mushrooms, stir and sauté for 5 minutes. Add the rest of the ingredients, toss, put the lid on and cook on High for 15 minutes. Release the pressure naturally for 10 minutes, divide the mix into bowls and serve for breakfast.

Nutrition: calories 23, fat 3.1, fiber 0.8, carbs 2.7, protein 1.5

Cinnamon Strawberry Oatmeal

Preparation time: 5 minutes | Cooking time: 10 minutes | Servings: 6

Ingredients:

- 2 cups almond milk
- ½ cup coconut cream
- 1 tablespoon cinnamon powder
- 1 cup coconut flakes
- 1 cup strawberries, halved

Directions:

In your instant pot, mix the almond milk with the rest of the ingredients, toss a bit, put the lid on and cook on High for 10 minutes. Release the pressure fast for 5 minutes, divide the mix into bowls and serve.

Nutrition: calories 285, fat 28.4, fiber 3.9, carbs 7.5, protein 2.9

Coconut Omelet

Preparation time: 10 minutes | Cooking time: 10 minutes | Servings: 4

Ingredients:

- 1 cup coconut flakes
- ½ cup coconut milk
- 4 eggs, whisked
- A pinch of salt and black pepper
- 1 tablespoon sweet paprika
- Cooking spray

Directions:

In a bowl, combine the eggs with the rest of the ingredients except the cooking spray and whisk really well. Grease the instant pot with the cooking spray, pour the omelet mix inside, spread, put the lid on and cook on High for 10 minutes. Release the pressure naturally for 10 minutes, divide the omelet between plates and serve.

Nutrition: calories 209, fat 18.6, fiber 3.1, carbs 6, protein 7.2

Leek Frittata

Preparation time: 10 minutes | Cooking time: 15 minutes | Servings: 4

Ingredients:

- 4 eggs, whisked
- 2 leeks, sliced
- 1 shallot, chopped
- 1 tablespoon sweet paprika
- A pinch of salt and black pepper
- 1 red bell pepper, chopped
- Cooking spray

Directions:

Grease your instant pot with the cooking spray, add leeks, shallot and the rest of the ingredients, toss, spread well into the pot, put the lid on and cooking on High for 15 minutes. Release the pressure naturally for 10 minutes, divide the frittata between plates and serve.

Nutrition: calories 106, fat 9.4, fiber 1.9, carbs 6.6, protein 6.8

Scallions and Peppers Bowls
Preparation time: 10 minutes | Cooking time: 15 minutes | Servings: 4

Ingredients:
- 1 red bell pepper, cut into strips
- 1 green bell pepper, cut into strips
- 3 garlic cloves, minced
- 4 scallions, chopped
- 2 teaspoons olive oil
- 2 tablespoons veggie stock
- 4 eggs, whisked
- 2 tablespoons red pepper sauce
- 1 tablespoon cilantro, chopped

Directions:
Set your instant pot on sauté mode, add the oil, heat it up, add the scallions and the garlic and cook for 2 minutes. Add the bell peppers and the rest of the ingredients, toss, put the lid on and cook on High for 10 minutes. Release the pressure naturally for 10 minutes, divide the mix into bowls and serve for breakfast.

Nutrition: calories 110, fat 6.9, fiber 1.3, carbs 6.7, protein 6.6

Curry Cauliflower Rice Bowls
Preparation time: 10 minutes | Cooking time: 12 minutes | Servings: 6

Ingredients:
- 1 broccoli head, florets separated
- 4 tomatoes, cubed
- 1 cup veggie stock
- 1 cup cauliflower rice
- 1 tablespoon ginger, grated
- 2 teaspoons curry powder
- 1 teaspoon chili flakes

Directions:
In your instant pot, mix the broccoli with the tomatoes and the rest of the ingredients, toss, put the lid on and cook on High for 12 minutes. Release the pressure naturally for 10 minutes, divide the mix into bowls and serve for breakfast.

Nutrition: calories 30, fat 5, fiber 2, carbs 4.5, protein 1.3

Ketogenic Instant Pot Lunch Recipes

Egg Salad

*Preparation time: 10 minutes | **Cooking time:** 5 minutes | **Servings:** 4*

Ingredients:

- 6 eggs
- 2 tablespoon avocado mayonnaise
- 2 cucumbers, sliced
- 1 avocado, peeled, pitted and cubed
- 2 spring onions, chopped
- 1 tablespoon cheddar cheese, grated
- 1 tablespoon mustard powder
- 1 tablespoon parsley, chopped
- A pinch of salt and black pepper
- 2 cups water

Directions:

Put the water in the instant pot, add the steamer basket and put the eggs inside. Put the lid on, cook on High for 5 minutes and then release the pressure naturally for 10. Cool the eggs down, peel, cut them into quarters and put them in a bowl. Add the cucumber, avocado and the rest of the ingredients, toss and serve for lunch.

Nutrition: calories 243, fat 18, fiber 4.8, carbs 8.7, protein 11.5

Green Beans and Rice Mix

*Preparation time: 10 minutes | **Cooking time:** 25 minutes | **Servings:** 4*

Ingredients:

- 1 shallot, chopped
- 1 red bell pepper, chopped
- 3 garlic cloves, minced
- 3 celery stalks, chopped
- 1 pound green beans, trimmed and halved
- A pinch of salt and black pepper
- 1 teaspoon hot sauce
- 1 tablespoon thyme, chopped
- 2 cups veggie stock
- 2 cups cauliflower rice

Directions:

In your instant pot, mix the shallot with the bell pepper and the rest of the ingredients, put the lid on and cook on High for 25 minutes. Release the pressure naturally for 10 minutes, divide the mix between plates and serve for lunch.

Nutrition: calories 52, fat 5.3, fiber 3.1, carbs 4.6, protein 2.7

Garlic Beef Mix

Preparation time: 10 minutes | Cooking time: 20 minutes | Servings: 6

Ingredients:

- 2 pounds beef, cubed
- 1 tablespoon olive oil
- ½ cup okra
- 3 spring onions, chopped
- A pinch of salt and black pepper
- 1 cup chicken stock
- 1 cup tomato passata
- 2 tablespoons mustard
- 1 cup cheddar cheese, shredded

Directions:

Set the instant pot on Sauté mode, add the oil, heat it up, add the meat and brown for 5 minutes. Add the rest of the ingredients except the cheese, put the lid on and cook on High for 15 minutes. Release the pressure naturally for 10 minutes, sprinkle the cheese on top, leave the mix aside for 10 minutes, divide it into bowls and serve.

Nutrition: calories 411, fat 19.3, fiber 1.6, carbs 5, protein 52.4

Parsley Beef Bowls

Preparation time: 10 minutes | Cooking time: 20 minutes | Servings: 6

Ingredients:

- 2 pounds beef roast, thinly sliced
- 1 tablespoon parsley, chopped
- 3 garlic cloves, minced
- A pinch of salt and black pepper
- ½ cup veggie stock
- 1 tablespoon lemon juice
- 2 tablespoons olive oil
- 1 teaspoon balsamic vinegar
- 1 cup feta cheese, crumbled

Directions:

Set the instant pot on Sauté mode, add the oil, heat it up, add the meat and garlic and brown for 5 minutes. Add salt, pepper and the rest of the ingredients except the cheese, put the lid on and cook on High for 15 minutes. Release the pressure naturally for 10 minutes, divide the mix into bowls, sprinkle the cheese on top and serve for lunch.

Nutrition: calories 390, fat 19.4, fiber 0.1, carbs 1.6, protein 9.5

Okra Soup

Preparation time: 10 minutes | Cooking time: 15 minutes | Servings: 4

Ingredients:

- 2 tablespoons olive oil
- 1 spring onion, chopped
- 3 cups okra
- 3 cups chicken stock
- 1 teaspoon garlic powder
- A pinch of salt and black pepper
- 1 cup cheddar cheese, shredded
- ½ cup coconut milk

Directions:

Set your instant pot on sauté mode, add the oil, heat it up, add the onion, stir and cook for 2 minutes. Add the rest of the ingredients, toss, put the lid on and cook on High for 13 minutes. Release the pressure naturally for 10 minutes, stir the soup again, divide it into bowls and serve.

Nutrition: calories 284, fat 24.1, fiber 3.2, carbs 7, protein 9.9

Greek Turkey and Sauce

Preparation time: 10 minutes | Cooking time: 25 minutes | Servings: 4

Ingredients:

- 1 turkey breast, skinless, boneless and cubed
- 1 tablespoon lime juice
- 1 cup Greek yogurt
- 1 cup tomato passata
- 1 tablespoon avocado oil
- 1 tablespoon garam masala
- ¼ teaspoon ginger, grated
- A pinch of salt and black pepper

Directions:

Set the instant pot on Sauté mode, add the oil, heat it up, add the turkey, ginger and garam masala, stir and brown for 5 minutes. Add the rest of the ingredients, toss, put the lid on and cook on High for 20 minutes. Release the pressure naturally for 10 minutes, divide the mix between plates and serve.

Nutrition: calories 20, fat 4.6, fiber 1.1, carbs 3.6, protein 0.9

Lime Pork Bowls

Preparation time: 10 minutes | Cooking time: 20 minutes | Servings: 6

Ingredients:
- 2 pounds pork stew meat, cubed
- 1 teaspoon garlic, minced
- 1 shallot, chopped
- 1 tablespoon beef stock
- 2 teaspoon lime juice
- ½ teaspoon chili powder
- 1 teaspoon sweet paprika
- ½ cup tomato passata
- 1 tablespoon olive oil
- A pinch of salt and black pepper

Directions:
Set your instant pot on sauté mode, add the oil, heat it up, add the shallot, garlic and the meat and brown for 5 minutes. Add the rest of the ingredients, put the lid on and cook on High for 15 minutes. Release the pressure naturally for 10 minutes, divide the mix between plates and serve.

Nutrition: calories 351, fat 17.1, fiber 0.6, carbs 2.4, protein 20

Coconut Broccoli Soup

Preparation time: 10 minutes | Cooking time: 15 minutes | Servings: 4

Ingredients:
- 1 broccoli head, florets separated
- 4 cups chicken stock
- A pinch of salt and white pepper
- ¼ teaspoon garlic powder
- 1 tablespoon chives, chopped
- 2 cups cheddar cheese, shredded
- 1 cup coconut cream

Directions:
In your instant pot, combine the broccoli with the stock and the rest of the ingredients except the cheese and the cream, stir, put the lid on and cook on High for 10 minutes. Release the pressure naturally for 10 minutes, set the pot on Sauté mode again, add the cheese and the cream, stir, blend using an immersion blender, cook for 5 minutes more, divide into bowls and serve.

Nutrition: calories 376, fat 33.5, fiber 1.4, carbs 4.9, protein 16.2

Pork Chops and Thyme Mushrooms
Preparation time: 10 minutes | Cooking time: 25 minutes | Servings: 4

Ingredients:
- 3 garlic cloves, minced
- 1 tablespoon olive oil
- 1 spring onion, chopped
- 10 white mushrooms, sliced
- 4 pork chops, bone-in
- 1 cup beef stock
- 1 tablespoon thyme, chopped
- 1 cup coconut cream

Directions:
Set your instant pot on sauté mode, add oil, heat it up, add the garlic and the mushrooms and sauté for 2 minutes. Add the meat and brown it for 2-3 minutes more. Add the rest of the ingredients, put the lid on and cook on High for 20 minutes. Release the pressure naturally for 10 minutes, divide everything between plates and serve.

Nutrition: calories 444, fat 38, fiber 2.2, carbs 6.3, protein 21.6

Mexican Pork and Okra Salad
Preparation time: 10 minutes | Cooking time: 30 minutes | Servings: 4

Ingredients:
- 2 pounds pork sirloin, cubed
- A pinch of salt and black pepper
- 2 teaspoons garlic powder
- 1 tablespoon olive oil
- 1 and ½ cups okra
- 1 cup tomato passata
- 2 garlic cloves, minced
- 1 tablespoon smoked paprika

Directions:
Set the instant pot on Sauté mode, add the oil, heat it up, add the meat, garlic, salt and pepper and brown for 5 minutes. Add the remaining ingredients, toss, put the lid on and cook on High for 25 minutes. Release the pressure naturally for 10 minutes, divide everything between plates and serve for lunch.

Nutrition: calories 66, fat 3.9, fiber 2, carbs 2.7, protein 1.6

Pork and Kale Meatballs
Preparation time: 10 minutes | Cooking time: 20 minutes | Servings: 6

Ingredients:
- 2 pounds pork stew meat, ground
- ¼ cup cheddar, grated
- 1 cup kale, chopped
- ¼ cup green onions, chopped
- 1 egg, whisked
- A pinch of salt and black pepper
- 1 tablespoon garlic, minced
- 1 tablespoon avocado oil
- 1 cup tomato passata
- ½ cup beef stock

Directions:
In a bowl, combine the meat with the cheese, kale, green onions, the egg, garlic, salt and pepper, stir well and shape medium meatballs out of this mix. Set the instant pot on Sauté mode, add the oil, heat it up, add the meatballs and brown them for 2 minutes on each side. Add the sauce and the stock, toss gently, put the lid on and cook on High for 15 minutes. Release the pressure naturally for 10 minutes, divide everything between plates and serve for lunch.

Nutrition: calories 362, fat 16.1, fiber 1, carbs 4.4, protein 26.7

Pork and Baby Spinach
Preparation time: 10 minutes | Cooking time: 20 minutes | Servings: 4

Ingredients:
- 1 pound pork stew meat, cubed
- 1 tablespoon olive oil
- ½ cup shallots, chopped
- 1 cup red bell peppers, chopped
- 2 garlic cloves, minced
- 1 cup beef stock
- 1 teaspoon chili powder
- 4 cups baby spinach

Directions:
Set your instant pot on sauté mode, add the oil, heat it up, add the meat and shallots and brown for 5 minutes. Add the rest of the ingredients except the spinach, put the lid on and cook on High for 10 minutes. Release the pressure naturally for 10 minutes, set the pot on Sauté mode again, add the spinach, toss, cook everything for 5 minutes more, divide between plates and serve.

Nutrition: calories 310, fat 14.9, fiber 1.3, carbs 7.6, protein 35.3

Cinnamon Turkey Curry

Preparation time: 10 minutes | Cooking time: 30 minutes | Servings: 4

Ingredients:

- 3 tomatoes, chopped
- 1 bug turkey breast, skinless, boneless and cubed
- 2 tablespoons avocado oil
- 1 cup chicken stock
- 14 ounces canned coconut milk
- 2 garlic cloves, minced
- 3 red chilies, chopped
- 1 tablespoon ginger, grated
- 1 teaspoon cinnamon, ground
- 1 teaspoon turmeric, ground
- 1 tablespoon lemon juice
- A pinch of salt and black pepper

Directions:

Set your instant pot on sauté mode, add the oil, heat it up, add the meat and brown for 5 minutes. Add the tomatoes and the rest of the ingredients, put the lid on and cook on High for 25 minutes. Release the pressure naturally for 10 minutes, divide everything between plates and serve.

Nutrition: calories 268, fat 25, fiber 4.3, carbs 7.9, protein 3.7

Basil Shrimp and Eggplants

Preparation time: 10 minutes | Cooking time: 10 minutes | Servings: 4

Ingredients:

- 2 eggplants, cubed
- 2 tablespoons veggie stock
- 2 tablespoons olive oil
- A pinch of salt and black pepper
- 4 garlic cloves, minced
- 1 pound shrimp, peeled and deveined
- Juice of 1 lime
- ½ teaspoon sweet paprika
- 2 tablespoons basil, chopped

Directions:

Set your instant pot on sauté mode, add the oil, heat it up, add the garlic and the eggplants and sauté for 2 minutes. Add the shrimp and the rest of the ingredients, put the lid on and cook on Low for 8 minutes. Release the pressure naturally for 10 minutes, divide everything into bowls and serve for lunch.

Nutrition: calories 269, fat 9.5, fiber 5.4, carbs 6.7, protein 28.8

Mushroom and Chicken Soup

Preparation time: 10 minutes | Cooking time: 20 minutes | Servings: 4

Ingredients:

- 1 shallot, chopped
- 1 quart chicken stock
- 1 pound mushrooms, sliced
- 1 tablespoon olive oil
- A pinch of salt and black pepper
- 2 tablespoons ginger, minced
- 1 pound chicken breast, skinless, boneless and cubed

Directions:

Set your instant pot on sauté mode, add the oil, heat it up, add the shallot and the mushrooms and cook for 4 minutes. Add the rest of the ingredients, put the lid on and cook on High for 15 minutes. Release the pressure naturally for 10 minutes, divide everything into bowls and serve.

Nutrition: calories 203, fat 7.4, fiber 1.5, carbs 6.4, protein 28.5

Cod and Tomato Passata

Preparation time: 10 minutes | Cooking time: 12 minutes | Servings: 4

Ingredients:

- 4 cod fillets, boneless and skinless
- A pinch of salt and black pepper
- 2 tablespoons chives, chopped
- 2 tablespoons olive oil
- 2 teaspoons lime juice
- 1 cup tomato passata
- 1 tablespoon basil, chopped

Directions:

Set your instant pot on sauté mode, add the oil, heat it up, add the cod and cook for 1 minute on each side. Add the rest of the ingredients, put the lid on and cook on High for 10 minutes. Release the pressure naturally for 10 minutes, divide everything between plates and serve.

Nutrition: calories 75, fat 7.1, fiber 1, carbs 3.4, protein 0.9

Chicken and Mustard Sauce

Preparation time: 10 minutes | Cooking time: 15 minutes | Servings: 4

Ingredients:

- 2 chicken breasts, skinless, boneless and halved
- 1 tablespoon olive oil
- Salt and black pepper to the taste
- ½ teaspoon onion powder
- ½ teaspoon garlic powder
- ½ cup chicken stock
- 1 teaspoon Dijon mustard
- 1 tablespoon basil, chopped

Directions:

Set your instant pot on sauté mode, add the oil, heat it up, add the chicken and brown for 2-3 minutes. Add the rest of the ingredients, put the lid on and cook on High for 12 minutes. Release the pressure naturally for 10 minutes, divide everything between plates and serve.

Nutrition: calories 34, fat 3.6, fiber 0.1, carbs 0.7, protein 0.3

Chicken and Avocado Mix

Preparation time: 10 minutes | Cooking time: 17 minutes | Servings: 8

Ingredients:

- 2 chicken breasts, skinless, boneless and halved
- 2 cups tomato passata
- A pinch of salt and black pepper
- 2 avocados, peeled, pitted and cubed
- 1 cup cheddar cheese, shredded
- 1 tablespoon olive oil

Directions:

Set your instant pot on sauté mode, add the oil, heat it up, add the chicken and brown for 5 minutes. Add the rest of the ingredients except the cheese and toss. Sprinkle the cheese on top, put the lid on and cook on High for 12 minutes. Release the pressure naturally for 10 minutes, divide everything between plates and serve.

Nutrition: calories 198, fat 16.4, fiber 4.6, carbs 6.6, protein 5.4

Tomato and Pork Soup

Preparation time: 10 minutes | Cooking time: 25 minutes | Servings: 4

Ingredients:

- 1 and ½ pounds pork stew meat, cubed
- 8 cups chicken stock
- 15 ounces tomatoes, chopped
- A pinch of salt and black pepper
- 1 tablespoon chives, chopped

Directions:

In your instant pot, mix all the ingredients except the chives, put the lid on and cook on High for 25 minutes. Release the pressure naturally for 10 minutes, divide the soup into bowls and serve.

Nutrition: calories 39, fat 4.3, fiber 1.2, carbs 3.4, protein 2.4

Cayenne Pork and Artichokes Stew

Preparation time: 10 minutes | Cooking time: 25 minutes | Servings: 4

Ingredients:

- 1 spring onion, chopped
- 2 and ½ pounds pork stew meat, cubed
- 15 ounces canned tomatoes, chopped
- 2 red chilies, chopped
- 1 and ½ cups canned artichoke hearts, chopped
- 2 garlic cloves, minced
- 2 tablespoons avocado oil
- 1 tablespoon cayenne pepper
- A pinch of salt and black pepper
- 1 teaspoon basil, dried

Directions:

Set your instant pot on sauté mode, add the oil, heat it up add the onion and the meat and brown for 5 minutes. Add the rest of the ingredients, put the lid on and cook on High for 20 minutes. Release the pressure naturally for 10 minutes, divide the stew into bowls and serve.

Nutrition: calories 36, fat 6.4, fiber 2.1, carbs 3.5, protein 1.4

Green Beans Soup

Preparation time: 10 minutes | Cooking time: 15 minutes | Servings: 4

Ingredients:

- 2 tablespoons olive oil
- 1 shallot, chopped
- 1 teaspoon garlic, minced
- 1 red bell pepper, chopped
- 8 cups chicken stock
- 1 and ½ pounds green beans, trimmed and halved
- 1 cup tomatoes, chopped
- 1 tablespoon chili powder
- 1 cup coconut cream

Directions:

Set your instant pot on sauté mode, add the oil, heat it up, add the shallot and the garlic and sauté for 2 minutes. Add the rest of the ingredients, put the lid on and cook on High for 13 minutes. Release the pressure naturally for 10 minutes, divide the soup into bowls and serve.

Nutrition: calories 242, fat 22.9, fiber 2.8, carbs 8.9, protein 3.7

Broccoli and Zucchini Soup

Preparation time: 10 minutes | Cooking time: 15 minutes | Servings: 4

Ingredients:

- 1 shallot, chopped
- 2 teaspoons avocado oil
- 1 pound broccoli florets
- 1 pound zucchinis, sliced
- 4 cups chicken stock
- 1 teaspoon basil, dried
- 1 tablespoon cilantro, chopped

Directions:

Set your instant pot on sauté mode, add the oil, heat it up, add the shallot and sauté for 2 minutes. Add the broccoli and the rest of the ingredients, put the lid on and cook on High for 12 minutes. Release the pressure naturally for 10 minutes, ladle the soup into bowls and serve.

Nutrition: calories 70, fat 11.3, fiber 4.3, carbs 6.7, protein 5.3

Beef Soup

Preparation time: 10 minutes | Cooking time: 25 minutes | Servings: 4

Ingredients:

- 1 and ½ pound beef meat, cubed
- 2 tablespoons olive oil
- A pinch of salt and black pepper
- 1 cup scallions, chopped
- 1 tablespoon sweet paprika
- 6 cups veggie stock
- 1 tablespoon parsley, chopped

Directions:

Set your instant pot on sauté mode, add the oil, heat it up, add the meat and the scallions and brown for 5 minutes. Add the rest of the ingredients, put the lid on and cook on High for 20 minutes. Release the pressure naturally for 10 minutes, ladle the soup into bowls and serve.

Nutrition: calories 73, fat 7.3, fiber 1.3, carbs 2.9, protein 0.8

Curry Tomato Cream

Preparation time: 10 minutes | Cooking time: 20 minutes | Servings: 4

Ingredients:

- 1 pound tomatoes, peeled and chopped
- A pinch of salt and black pepper
- 3 garlic cloves, minced
- 1 tablespoon cilantro, chopped
- 2 cups coconut cream
- 2 cups chicken stock
- 1 tablespoon red curry paste
- 2 tablespoons chives, chopped

Directions:

In your instant pot, combine the tomatoes with salt, pepper, garlic and the stock, put the lid on and cook on High for 20 minutes. Release the pressure naturally for 10 minutes, transfer the soup to a blender, add the cream and curry paste, pulse well, divide into bowls and serve with the chives and cilantro sprinkled on top.

Nutrition: calories 320, fat 30.2, fiber 4.1, carbs 8.1, protein 4.2

Spinach Soup

Preparation time: 10 minutes | Cooking time: 20 minutes | Servings: 4

Ingredients:

- 2 teaspoons olive oil
- 1 scallion, chopped
- 1 celery stalk, chopped
- 4 cups baby spinach
- 4 garlic cloves, minced
- 2 teaspoons cumin, ground
- 6 cups veggie stock
- 1 teaspoon basil, dried

Directions:

Set your instant pot on sauté mode, add the oil, heat it up, add the scallion and garlic and sauté for 5 minutes. Add the celery, cumin and the basil and sauté for 4 minutes more. Add the spinach and the stock, put the lid on and cook on High for 10 minutes. Release the pressure naturally for 10 minutes, ladle the soup into bowls and serve.

Nutrition: calories 37, fat 3.1, fiber 1, carbs 3, protein 1.4

Cabbage Soup

Preparation time: 6 minutes | Cooking time: 15 minutes | Servings: 4

Ingredients:

- 1 shallot, chopped
- 1 pound green cabbage, shredded
- 12 cups chicken stock
- 1 celery stalk, chopped
- 1 tablespoon olive oil
- A pinch of salt and black pepper
- 2 tablespoons dill, chopped

Directions:

Set your instant pot on sauté mode, add oil, heat it up, add the shallot and sauté for 2 minutes. Add the rest of the ingredients, put the lid on and cook on High for 13 minutes. Release the pressure fast for 6 minutes, ladle the soup into bowls and serve.

Nutrition: calories 92, fat 5.4, fiber 3.1, carbs 5.7, protein 3.9

Cheesy Coconut Cream

Preparation time: 5 minutes | Cooking time: 20 minutes | Servings: 4

Ingredients:

- 2 tablespoons olive oil
- ½ cup spring onions, chopped
- 6 cups chicken stock
- A pinch of salt and black pepper
- 2 tablespoons parsley, chopped
- 2 cups coconut cream
- 1 cup cheddar cheese, grated

Directions:

Set your instant pot on Sauté mode, add the oil, heat it up, add the spring onions and sauté for 2-3 minutes. Add the rest of the ingredients, whisk, put the lid on and cook on High for 15 minutes. Release the pressure naturally for 10 minutes, divide the soup into bowls and serve.

Nutrition: calories 313, fat 30.5, fiber 2, carbs 6.1, protein 7.4

Eggplant Soup

Preparation time: 10 minutes | Cooking time: 15 minutes | Servings: 4

Ingredients:

- 1 tablespoon avocado oil
- 1 celery stalk, chopped
- 1 shallot chopped
- 3 eggplants, cubed
- 2 tomatoes, chopped
- 8 cups chicken stock
- A pinch of salt and black pepper
- 2 tablespoons rosemary, chopped

Directions:

Set your instant pot on Sauté mode, add the oil, heat it up, add the shallot and celery, stir and sauté for 3 minutes. Add the eggplants and the rest of the ingredients, put the lid on and cook on High for 12 minutes. Release the pressure naturally for 10 minutes, ladle the soup into bowls and serve.

Nutrition: calories 144, fat 5.7, fiber 0.2, carbs 5.3, protein 6.1

Bell Pepper Cream

Preparation time: 10 minutes | Cooking time: 20 minutes | Servings: 4

Ingredients:

- 1 shallot, chopped
- 2 tablespoons olive oil
- 4 red bell peppers, roughly chopped
- 2 tomatoes, cubed
- 3 tablespoons tomato paste
- 6 cups chicken stock
- ½ teaspoon red pepper flakes
- 1 teaspoon chives, chopped

Directions:

Set the instant pot on Sauté mode, add the oil, heat it up, add the shallot and cook for 2 minutes Add the rest of the ingredients except the chives, put the lid on and cook on High for 18 minutes. Release the pressure naturally for 10 minutes, blend the soup using an immersion blender, divide it into bowls and serve.

Nutrition: calories 134, fat 8.4, fiber 2.8, carbs 5.4, protein 3.3

Chicken and Asparagus Soup

Preparation time: 10 minutes | Cooking time: 20 minutes | Servings: 4

Ingredients:

- 1 asparagus stalk, trimmed and halved
- A pinch of salt and black pepper
- 2 chicken breasts, skinless, boneless and cubed
- 2 scallions, chopped
- 1 tablespoon avocado oil
- 1 tablespoon sweet chili sauce
- ¼ cup parsley, chopped
- 5 cups chicken stock

Directions:

Set the instant pot on Sauté mode, add the oil, heat it up, add the scallions and the chili sauce and cook for 3 minutes. Add the chicken and brown for 2 minutes more. Add the rest of the ingredients, put the lid on and cook on High for 15 minutes. Release the pressure naturally for 10 minutes, ladle the soup into bowls and serve.

Nutrition: calories 108, fat 4.4, fiber 0.5, carbs 3.1, protein 1.1

Hot Cod Stew

Preparation time: 5 minutes | Cooking time: 12 minutes | Servings: 4

Ingredients:

- 1 pound cod fillets, boneless, skinless and cubed
- 1 cup chicken stock
- 1 tablespoon hot sauce
- 1 tablespoon hot paprika
- A pinch of salt and black pepper
- 1 tablespoon cilantro, chopped

Directions:

In your instant pot, combine the cod with the rest of the ingredients, put the lid on and cook on High for 12 minutes. Release the pressure fast for 5 minutes, divide the stew into bowls and serve.

Nutrition: calories 100, fat 4.3, fiber 1, carbs 3.2, protein 1.4

Lamb Stew

Preparation time: 10 minutes | Cooking time: 30 minutes | Servings: 4

Ingredients:

- 1 tablespoon avocado oil
- 1 and ½ pound lamb shoulder, cubed
- 1 cup black olives, pitted and sliced
- 2 tomatoes, cubed
- A pinch of salt and black pepper
- 1 cup beef stock
- 1 cup tomato passata
- 2 tablespoons basil, chopped

Directions:

Set your instant pot on Sauté mode, add the oil, heat it up, add the meat and brown for 5 minutes. Add the rest of the ingredients except the basil, put the lid on and cook on High for 25 minutes. Release the pressure naturally for 10 minutes, divide the stew into bowls and serve with the basil, sprinkled on top.

Nutrition: calories 251, fat 5.6, fiber 2.7, carbs 4.7, protein 8.3

Shrimp and Olives Stew

Preparation time: 10 minutes | Cooking time: 10 minutes | Servings: 4

Ingredients:

- 1 and ½ pounds shrimp, peeled and deveined
- 1 cup black olives, pitted and halved
- 2 tablespoons olive oil
- 2 scallions, chopped
- 2 tomatoes, cubed
- 1 tablespoon sweet paprika
- ½ cup chicken stock

Directions:

Set your instant pot on Sauté mode, add the oil, heat it up, add the scallions and cook for 2 minutes. Add the rest of the ingredients, put the lid on and cook on Low for 8 minutes. Release the pressure naturally for 10 minutes, divide the stew into bowls and serve.

Nutrition: calories 118, fat 11, fiber 2.7, carbs 6.1, protein 1.3

Turkey Stew

Preparation time: 10 minutes | Cooking time: 20 minutes | Servings: 4

Ingredients:

- 1 turkey breast, skinless, boneless and cubed
- 1 teaspoon olive oil
- A pinch of salt and black pepper
- 1 tablespoon avocado oil
- 1 celery stalk, chopped
- 2 cups chicken stock
- 2 cups tomatoes, chopped
- 1 tablespoons cilantro, chopped

Directions:

Set your instant pot on Sauté mode, add the oil, heat it up, add the meat and cook for 5 minutes. Add the rest of the ingredients, put the lid on and cook on High for 15 minutes. Release the pressure naturally for 10 minutes, divide the stew into bowls and serve.

Nutrition: calories 81, fat 4.3, fiber 1.5, carbs 6, protein 8.6

Kale Stew

Preparation time: 10 minutes | Cooking time: 20 minutes | Servings: 4

Ingredients:

- 1 shallot, chopped
- 2 garlic cloves, minced
- 1 pound kale, torn
- 20 ounces canned tomatoes, chopped
- 2 tablespoons olive oil
- A pinch of salt and black pepper
- ½ teaspoon cayenne pepper
- 1 tablespoon parsley, chopped

Directions:

Set the instant pot on Sauté mode, add the oil, heat it up, add the shallot and garlic and cook for 2 minutes. Add the other ingredients, put the lid on and cook on High for 18 minutes. Release the pressure naturally for 10 minutes, divide the stew into bowls and serve.

Nutrition: calories 145, fat 7.3, fiber 3.5, carbs 5.2, protein 4.8

Turmeric Cabbage Stew

Preparation time: 10 minutes | Cooking time: 20 minutes | Servings: 4

Ingredients:

- 3 garlic cloves, chopped
- 1 celery stalk, chopped
- 2 cups green cabbage, shredded
- 1 cup veggie stock
- ½ tablespoon avocado oil
- 14 ounces canned tomatoes, chopped
- A pinch of salt and black pepper
- 1 teaspoon turmeric powder

Directions:

Set your instant pot on Sauté mode, add the oil, heat it up, add the celery and garlic and sauté for 2 minutes. Add the rest of the ingredients, put the lid on and cook on High for 15 minutes. Release the pressure naturally for 10 minutes, divide the stew into bowls and serve.

Nutrition: calories 35, fat 4.2, fiber 2.4, carbs 3.2, protein 1.6

Chili Mushrooms Stew

Preparation time: 10 minutes | Cooking time: 15 minutes | Servings: 4

Ingredients:

- 2 spring onions, chopped
- 2 teaspoons avocado oil
- 2 garlic cloves, minced
- 1 teaspoon chili powder
- A pinch of salt and black pepper
- 6 cups mushrooms, sliced
- 2 cups veggie stock
- 1 cup tomato passata
- 1 tablespoon chives, chopped

Directions:

Set your instant pot on Sauté mode, add the oil, heat it up, add the onions and the garlic and sauté for 2 minutes. Add the mushrooms and sauté for 2 minutes more. Add the rest of the ingredients except the cilantro, put the lid on and cook on High for 10 minutes. Release the pressure naturally for 10 minutes, divide the stew into bowls and serve with the chives sprinkled on top.

Nutrition: calories 56, fat 4.5, fiber 2.2, carbs 3.7, protein 4.7

Zucchini and Lamb Stew

Preparation time: 10 minutes | Cooking time: 30 minutes | Servings: 4

Ingredients:

- 2 tablespoons olive oil
- 2 zucchinis, sliced
- A pinch of salt and black pepper
- 1 pound lamb shoulder, cubed
- 2 tablespoons tomato passata
- ¼ cup veggie stock
- 1 teaspoon sweet paprika
- 1 tablespoon dill, chopped

Directions:

Set your instant pot on Sauté mode, add the oil, heat it up, the meat and brown for 5 minutes. Add the rest of the ingredients, put the lid on and cook on High for 25 minutes. Release the pressure naturally for 10 minutes, divide the stew into bowls and serve.

Nutrition: calories 292, fat 15.6, fiber 1.5, carbs 4.5, protein 33.4

Beef and Cauliflower Stew

Preparation time: 10 minutes | Cooking time: 25 minutes | Servings: 4

Ingredients:

- 1 tablespoon olive oil
- 2 shallots, chopped
- A pinch of salt and black pepper
- 1 pound beef stew meat, cubed
- 15 ounces canned tomatoes, chopped
- 5 cups chicken stock
- 1 tablespoon cilantro, chopped

Directions:

Set your instant pot on Sauté mode, add the oil, heat it up, add the shallot and the meat and brown for 5 minutes. Add the rest of the ingredients, put the lid on and cook on High for 20 minutes.. Release the pressure naturally for 10 minutes, divide the stew into bowls and serve.

Nutrition: calories 272, fat 11.5, fiber 1.3, carbs 5.1, protein 35.6

Chicken and Brussels Sprouts Stew

Preparation time: 10 minutes | Cooking time: 25 minutes | Servings: 4

Ingredients:

- 1 tablespoon avocado oil
- 2 scallions, chopped
- 1 pound chicken breasts, skinless, boneless and cubed
- ½ pound Brussels sprouts, halved
- 1 teaspoon basil, chopped
- 1 and ½ cups chicken stock
- A pinch of salt and black pepper
- 1 tablespoon tomato paste

Directions:

Set your instant pot on Sauté mode, add the oil, heat it up, add the scallions and the chicken and brown for 5 minutes. Add the remaining ingredients, put the lid on and cook on High for 20 minutes. Release the pressure naturally for 10 minutes, divide the stew into bowls and serve.

Nutrition: calories 250, fat 9.1, fiber 2.7, carbs 6.7, protein 35.1

Cod and Shrimp Stew

Preparation time: 5 minutes | Cooking time: 14 minutes | Servings: 4

Ingredients:

- 1 and ½ pounds shrimp, peeled and deveined
- 1 and ½ pounds cod fillets, boneless, skinless and cubed
- 20 ounces canned tomatoes, chopped
- 3 garlic cloves, minced
- 2 tablespoons parsley, chopped
- 2 cups veggie stock
- 1 tablespoon basil, dried
- A pinch of salt and black pepper

Directions:

In your instant pot, mix the shrimp with the cod and the rest of the ingredients, put the lid on and cook on High for 14 minutes. Release the pressure fast for 5 minutes, divide the stew into bowls and serve.

Nutrition: calories 130, fat 7.5, fiber 1.8, carbs 6.4, protein 1.5

Beef Meatballs Stew

Preparation time: 10 minutes | Cooking time: 15 minutes | Servings: 4

Ingredients:

- 1 and ½ pounds beef meat, ground
- 1 egg
- 2 tablespoons cilantro, chopped
- 2 garlic cloves, minced
- A pinch of salt and black pepper
- ¾ cup beef stock
- ½ cup tomato passata
- ½ teaspoon sweet paprika
- 2 tablespoons olive oil
- 1 tablespoon parsley, chopped

Directions:

In a bowl, mix the beef with the egg, salt, pepper, garlic and the cilantro, stir and shape medium meatballs out of this mix. Set the instant pot on Sauté mode, add the oil, heat it up, add the meatballs and brown for 2 minutes on each side. Add the rest of the ingredients, put the lid on and cook on High for 10 minutes. Release the pressure naturally for 10 minutes, divide the mix between plates and serve.

Nutrition: calories 90, fat 8.3, fiber 0.6, carbs 2.5, protein 2.4

Salmon Stew

Preparation time: 10 minutes | Cooking time: 15 minutes | Servings: 4

Ingredients:

- 4 salmon fillets, boneless and cubed
- 2 cups chicken stock
- 2 tablespoons olive oil
- 2 shallots, chopped
- 2 tomatoes, cubed
- 1 tablespoon sweet paprika
- ½ teaspoon chili powder
- 1 zucchini, chopped
- 1 eggplant, chopped
- A pinch of salt and black pepper

Directions:

Set the instant pot on Sauté mode, add the oil, heat it up, add the shallots and cook for 2 minutes. Add the salmon and the rest of the ingredients, put the lid on and cook on High for 13 minutes. Release the pressure naturally for 10 minutes, divide the stew into bowls and serve.

Nutrition: calories 354, fat 19, fiber 6.1, carbs 7.6, protein 34.2

Veggie Soup

Preparation time: 10 minutes | Cooking time: 15 minutes | Servings: 4

Ingredients:

- 1 tablespoon avocado oil
- 1 celery stalk, chopped
- 2 tomatoes, chopped
- 1 shallot, chopped
- 1 zucchini, chopped
- 2 garlic cloves, minced
- 6 cups chicken stock
- A pinch of salt and black pepper
- 1 teaspoon basil, dried
- 2 cups kale, chopped
- 2 tablespoons basil, chopped

Directions:

Set your instant pot on Sauté mode, add oil, heat it up, add the shallot and the garlic and sauté for 2 minutes. Add the rest of the ingredients except the basil, put the lid on and cook on High for 13 minutes. Release the pressure naturally for 10 minutes, ladle into bowls and serve with the basil sprinkled on top.

Nutrition: calories 58, fat 3.1, fiber 1.2, carbs 2.4, protein 3.4

Artichokes Cream

Preparation time: 10 minutes | Cooking time: 15 minutes | Servings: 4

Ingredients:

- 2 cups artichoke hearts, chopped
- 3 tablespoons ghee
- 6 cups chicken stock
- 1 shallot, chopped
- ¼ teaspoon lime juice
- 1 teaspoon rosemary, dried
- ½ cup coconut cream
- A pinch of salt and black pepper

Directions:

Set your instant pot on Sauté mode, add the ghee, heat it up, add the shallot and cook for 2 minutes. Add the rest of the ingredients, put the lid on and cook on High for 13 minutes. Release the pressure naturally for 10 minutes, blend the soup using an immersion blender, ladle into bowls and serve.

Nutrition: calories 169, fat 17.6, fiber 0.3, carbs 3, protein 1.8

Leek Soup

Preparation time: 10 minutes | Cooking time: 15 minutes | Servings: 4

Ingredients:

- 4 cups chicken stock
- 2 leeks, chopped
- 1 tablespoon olive oil
- 1 shallot, minced
- 1 tablespoon sweet paprika
- 1 tablespoon tomato paste
- A pinch of salt and black pepper
- 1 tablespoon cilantro, chopped

Directions:

Set the instant pot on Sauté mode, add the oil, heat it up, add the shallot and the leeks and sauté for 2 minutes. Add the rest of the ingredients, put the lid on and cook on High for 13 minutes. Release the pressure naturally for 10 minutes, ladle the soup into bowls and serve.

Nutrition: calories 75, fat 4.4, fiber 1.6, carbs 3.4, protein 1.8

Sage Chicken and Turkey Stew

Preparation time: 10 minutes | Cooking time: 25 minutes | Servings: 4

Ingredients:

- ½ pound turkey breast, skinless, boneless and cubed
- ½ pound chicken breast, skinless, boneless and cubed
- 1 tablespoon sage, chopped
- 1 teaspoon olive oil
- ¼ pound tomatoes, cubed
- 1 shallot, chopped
- A pinch of salt and black pepper
- 2 tablespoons tomato paste
- 2 and ½ cups chicken stock
- 1 tablespoon cilantro, chopped

Directions:

Set your instant pot on Sauté mode, add oil, heat it up, add the turkey, chicken and the shallots, and brown for 5 minutes. Add the rest of the ingredients except the cilantro, put the lid on and cook on High for 20 minutes. Release the pressure naturally for 10 minutes, divide the stew into bowls, sprinkle the cilantro on top and serve.

Nutrition: calories 147, fat 3.7, fiber 1.2, carbs 2.5, protein 22.4

Bell Peppers and Kale Soup

Preparation time: 10 minutes | Cooking time: 15 minutes | Servings: 4

Ingredients:

- 4 red bell peppers, deseeded and roughly chopped
- ½ pound kale, torn
- A pinch of salt and black pepper
- 1 cup tomato passata
- 4 cups chicken stock
- 1 tablespoon cilantro, chopped

Directions:

In your instant pot, mix the bell peppers with the kale and the rest of the ingredients, put the lid on and cook on High for 15 minutes. Release the pressure naturally for 10 minutes, ladle the soup into bowls and serve.

Nutrition: calories 100, fat 6.3, fiber 2.2, carbs 3.7, protein 21.2

Tomato and Olives Stew

Preparation time: 5 minutes | Cooking time: 15 minutes | Servings: 4

Ingredients:

- 1 pound tomatoes, cubed
- 1 tablespoon olive oil
- A pinch of salt and black pepper
- 1 cup kalamata olives, pitted
- 1 teaspoon thyme, dried
- 1 cup chicken stock
- 1 tablespoon oregano, chopped

Directions:

Set your instant pot on Sauté mode, add the oil, heat it up, add the tomatoes and cook them for 2 minutes. Add the rest of the ingredients except the oregano, put the lid on and cook on High for 15 minutes Release the pressure fast for 5 minutes, add the oregano, stir, divide the stew into bowls and serve right away.

Nutrition: calories 96, fat 7.6, fiber 3, carbs 6.8, protein 1.6

Creamy Brussels Sprouts Stew

Preparation time: 5 minutes | Cooking time: 25 minutes | Servings: 4

Ingredients:

- 1 tablespoon olive oil
- 2 shallots, chopped
- 1 pound Brussels sprouts, halved
- A pinch of salt and black pepper
- 1 cup chicken stock
- 1 cup coconut cream
- 1 tablespoon chives, chopped

Directions:

Set your instant pot on Sauté mode, add the oil, heat it up, add the shallots and sauté for 5 minutes. Add the rest of the ingredients except the chives, put the lid on and cook on High for 20 minutes. Release the pressure fast for 5 minutes, add the chives, stir the stew, divide it into bowls and serve.

Nutrition: calories 220, fat 16.7, fiber 5.6, carbs 6.8, protein 5.4

Ketogenic Instant Pot Side Dish Recipes

Ginger Cabbage and Radish Mix
Preparation time: 10 minutes | Cooking time: 15 minutes | Servings: 4

Ingredients:
- 1 red cabbage head, shredded
- 2 tablespoons veggie stock
- 1 cup radish, sliced
- 3 garlic cloves, minced
- 1 tablespoon coconut aminos
- 1 tablespoon olive oil
- ½ inch ginger, grated

Directions:

Set the instant pot on Sauté mode, add the oil, heat it up, add the garlic and the ginger and sauté for 3 minutes. Add the rest of the ingredients, put the lid on and cook on High for 12 minutes. Release the pressure naturally for 10 minutes, divide the mix between plates and serve as a side dish.

Nutrition: calories 83, fat 4.4, fiber 2.1, carbs 3.3, protein 2.6

Chives Brussels Sprouts
Preparation time: 10 minutes | Cooking time: 10 minutes | Servings: 4

Ingredients:
- 1 pound Brussels sprouts, halved
- ¼ cup chicken stock
- A pinch of salt and black pepper
- 1 tablespoon green onions, chopped
- 2 tablespoons olive oil
- 1 tablespoon tomato passata
- 1 tablespoon chives, chopped

Directions:

In your instant pot, combine the sprouts with the stock and the rest of the ingredients, put the lid on and cook on High for 10 minutes. Release the pressure naturally for 10 minutes, divide the mix between plates and serve as a side dish.

Nutrition: calories 112, fat 7.5, fiber 2.4, carbs 4.5, protein 4

Mozzarella Broccoli
Preparation time: 10 minutes | Cooking time: 10 minutes | Servings: 4

Ingredients:
- 1 pound broccoli florets
- ½ cup veggie stock
- 2 shallots, chopped
- A pinch of salt and black pepper
- 1 cup mozzarella, shredded
- 1 tablespoon cilantro, chopped
- 3 tablespoons olive oil

Directions:
Set the instant pot on Sauté mode, add the oil, heat it up, add the shallots and sauté for 2 minutes. Add the rest of the ingredients except the mozzarella and toss. Sprinkle the mozzarella on top, put the lid on and cook on High for 8 minutes. Release the pressure naturally for 10 minutes, divide the mix between plates and serve.

Nutrition: calories 149, fat 12.1, fiber 3, carbs 7.8, protein 5.2

Garlic Broccoli Mix
Preparation time: 10 minutes | Cooking time: 15 minutes | Servings: 4

Ingredients:
- 2 tablespoons ghee, melted
- 3 garlic cloves, minced
- 1 pound broccoli florets
- ½ cup coconut cream
- 3 tablespoons lime juice
- 1 tablespoon dill, chopped
- ½ cup chicken stock
- A pinch of salt and black pepper

Directions:
Set your instant pot on sauté mode, add the ghee, heat it up, add the garlic and cook for 2 minutes. Add the broccoli and the rest of the ingredients, toss, put the lid on and cook on High for 12 minutes. Release the pressure naturally for 10 minutes, divide the mix between plates and serve.

Nutrition: calories 170, fat 14, fiber 3.8, carbs 6.5, protein 4.3

Balsamic Mushroom and Radish Mix

Preparation time: 10 minutes | Cooking time: 15 minutes | Servings: 4

Ingredients:

- 2 tablespoons avocado oil
- A pinch of salt and black pepper
- 1 pound white mushrooms, sliced
- ¼ cup chicken stock
- 1 cup radishes, sliced
- 2 tablespoons balsamic vinegar
- 1 tablespoon parsley, chopped

Directions:

Set the instant pot on sauté mode, add the oil, heat it up, add the mushrooms and sauté for 5 minutes. Add the rest of the ingredients, put the lid on and cook on High for 10 minutes. Release the pressure naturally for 10 minutes, divide the mix between plates and serve.

Nutrition: calories 41, fat 4.3, fiber 1.9, carbs 3.5, protein 3.9

Collard Greens and Tomatoes

Preparation time: 10 minutes | Cooking time: 15 minutes | Servings: 4

Ingredients:

- 2 tablespoons avocado oil
- 1 pound collard greens
- ¼ cup chicken stock
- 1 tablespoon lime juice
- 2 cups cherry tomatoes, chopped
- 2 spring onions, chopped
- A pinch of salt and black pepper
- 1 tablespoon chives, chopped

Directions:

Set your instant pot on sauté mode, add the oil, heat it up, add the onions and sauté for 2 minutes. Add the rest of the ingredients, put the lid on and cook on High for 13 minutes. Release the pressure naturally for 10 minutes, divide the mix between plates and serve.

Nutrition: calories 60, fat 4.6, fiber 1.4, carbs 3.2, protein 3.6

Balsamic Spinach

Preparation time: 5 minutes | Cooking time: 7 minutes | Servings: 4

Ingredients:

- ¼ cup veggie stock
- 1 and ½ pound baby spinach
- 1 tablespoon balsamic vinegar
- 1 tablespoon walnuts, chopped
- 1 tablespoon chives, chopped

Directions:

In your instant pot, mix the spinach with the stock and the rest of the ingredients, put the lid on and cook on High for 7 minutes. Release the pressure fast for 5 minutes, divide the mix between plates and serve.

Nutrition: calories 13, fat 1.2, fiber 0.2, carbs 0.3, protein 0.5

Paprika Mushrooms

Preparation time: 10 minutes | Cooking time: 15 minutes | Servings: 4

Ingredients:

- and ½ pound white mushrooms, sliced
- A pinch of salt and black pepper
- 1 tablespoon sweet paprika
- 1 cup veggie stock
- 1 tablespoon dill, chopped
- 1 tablespoon rosemary, chopped
- 1 tablespoon avocado oil

Directions:

Set your instant pot on sauté mode, add the oil, heat it up, add the mushrooms and sauté them for 5 minutes. Add the rest of the ingredients, put the lid on and cook on High for 10 minutes. Release the pressure naturally for 10 minutes, divide the mix between plates and serve.

Nutrition: calories 14, fat 2.3, fiber 1.3, carbs 2.1, protein 0.5

Coconut Spinach Mix

Preparation time: 5 minutes | Cooking time: 7 minutes | Servings: 4

Ingredients:

- 1 and ½ pounds baby spinach
- ¼ cup coconut cream
- 1 tablespoon chili powder
- A pinch of salt and black pepper
- 1 tablespoon cilantro, chopped

Directions:

In your instant pot, combine the spinach with the rest of the ingredients, put the lid on and cook on High for 7 minutes. Release the pressure fast for 5 minutes, divide the mix between plates and serve as a side dish.

Nutrition: calories 41, fat 3.9, fiber 1, carbs 1.9, protein 0.6

Chili Eggplant and Collard Greens

Preparation time: 10 minutes | Cooking time: 15 minutes | Servings: 4

Ingredients:

- 1 big eggplant, cubed
- 1 pound collard greens, halved
- 2 tablespoons avocado oil
- 2 teaspoons chili paste
- ½ cup chicken stock
- 1 tablespoon cilantro, chopped
- 4 green onions, chopped

Directions:

Set your instant pot on sauté mode, add the oil, heat it up, add the spring onions and the eggplants, stir and cook for 4 minutes. Add the rest of the ingredients, put the lid on and cook on High for 10 minutes. Release the pressure naturally for 10 minutes, divide everything between plates and serve.

Nutrition: calories 84, fat 2.4, fiber 2, carbs 6, protein 4.2

Chard and Mushrooms Mix

Preparation time: 10 minutes | Cooking time: 12 minutes | Servings: 4

Ingredients:

- 2 tablespoons olive oil
- 1 pound white mushrooms, sliced
- 1 red chard bunch, roughly chopped
- ¼ cup chicken stock
- 1 teaspoon garlic powder
- A pinch of salt and black pepper
- 3 tablespoons parsley, chopped

Directions:

Set your instant pot on sauté mode, add the oil, heat it up, add the mushrooms and sauté for 2 minutes. Add the rest of the ingredients, put the lid on and cook on High for 10 minutes. Release the pressure naturally for 10 minutes, divide the mix between plates and serve as a side dish.

Nutrition: calories 88, fat 7.4, fiber 1.3, carbs 4.5, protein 3.8

Creamy Cauliflower

Preparation time: 10 minutes | Cooking time: 15 minutes | Servings: 4

Ingredients:

- 1 pound cauliflower florets
- 1 cup red onion, chopped
- ¼ cup chicken stock
- A pinch of salt and black pepper
- 2 tablespoons balsamic vinegar
- 1 cup coconut cream

Directions:

In your instant pot, mix the cauliflower with the rest of the ingredients, put the lid on and cook on High for 15 minutes. Release the pressure naturally for 10 minutes, divide the mix between plates and serve.

Nutrition: calories 180, fat 14.5, fiber 4.5, carbs 7.5, protein 4

Creamy Green Beans

Preparation time: 10 minutes | Cooking time: 15 minutes | Servings: 4

Ingredients:

- 10 ounces green beans, trimmed and halved
- A pinch of salt and black pepper
- 1/3 cup parmesan, grated
- 2 ounces cream cheese
- 1/3 cup coconut cream
- 1 tablespoon dill, chopped

Directions:

In your instant pot, mix the green beans with the cream cheese and the rest of the ingredients, put the lid on and cook on High for 15 minutes. Release the pressure naturally for 10 minutes, divide the mix between plates and serve as a side dish.

Nutrition: calories 119, fat 9.8, fiber 3, carbs 6, protein 3

Spinach and Radish Mix

Preparation time: 5 minutes | Cooking time: 7 minutes | Servings: 4

Ingredients:

- 1 pound spinach, torn
- 2 cups radishes, sliced
- A pinch of salt and black pepper
- ¼ cup veggie stock
- 1 teaspoon chili powder
- 1 tablespoon parsley, chopped

Directions:

In your instant pot, mix the spinach with the radishes and the rest of the ingredients, put the lid on and cook on High for 7 minutes. Release the pressure fast for 5 minutes, divide the mix between plates and serve.

Nutrition: calories 70, fat 4.4, fiber 3.7, carbs 4, protein 3.7

Lemon Cabbage Mix

Preparation time: 10 minutes | Cooking time: 10 minutes | Servings: 4

Ingredients:

- 1 pound green cabbage, shredded
- ½ cup chicken stock
- A pinch of salt and black pepper
- 1 tablespoon lemon juice
- 1 tablespoon chives, chopped
- 1 tablespoon lemon zest, grated

Directions:

In your instant pot, mix the cabbage with the stock and the rest of the ingredients, put the lid on and cook on High for 10 minutes. Release the pressure naturally for 10 minutes, divide the mix between plates sand serve.

Nutrition: calories 34, fat 2.4, fiber 1, carbs 1.9, protein 1.6

Herbed Radish Mix

Preparation time: 10 minutes | Cooking time: 12 minutes | Servings: 4

Ingredients:

- 3 cups red radishes, halved
- ½ cup veggie stock
- 2 tablespoons basil, chopped
- 1 tablespoon oregano, chopped
- 1 tablespoon chives, chopped
- 1 tablespoon green onion, chopped
- A pinch of salt and black pepper

Directions:

In your instant pot, combine the radishes with the stock and the rest of the ingredients, put the lid on and cook on High for 12 minutes. Release the pressure naturally for 10 minutes, divide the mix between plates and serve.

Nutrition: calories 30, fat 1.3, fiber 0.1, carbs 1, protein 0.8

Asparagus Mix

Preparation time: 5 minutes | Cooking time: 8 minutes | Servings: 4

Ingredients:

- 1 pound asparagus, trimmed and halved
- 2 teaspoons mustard
- ¼ cup coconut cream
- 2 garlic cloves, minced
- 1 tablespoon chives, chopped
- Salt and black pepper to the taste

Directions:

In your instant pot, combine the asparagus with the rest of the ingredients, put the lid on and cook on High for 8 minutes. Release the pressure fast for 5 minutes, divide the mix between plates and serve.

Nutrition: calories 67, fat 4.2, fiber 3, carbs 3.9, protein 3.4

Pine Nuts Savoy Cabbage

Preparation time: 10 minutes | Cooking time: 15 minutes | Servings: 4

Ingredients:

- 1 Savoy cabbage, shredded
- 2 tablespoons avocado oil
- 1 tablespoon balsamic vinegar
- ¼ cup pine nuts, toasted
- ½ cup veggie stock
- Salt and black pepper to the taste

Directions:

Set your instant pot on sauté mode, add the oil, heat it up, add the cabbage and sauté for 2 minutes. Add the rest of the ingredients, put the lid on and cook on High for 15 minutes. Release the pressure naturally for 10 minutes, divide the mix between plates and serve as a side dish.

Nutrition: calories 67, fat 6.7, fiber 0.5, carbs 1.5, protein 1.3

Spinach and Fennel Mix

Preparation time: 10 minutes | Cooking time: 10 minutes | Servings: 4

Ingredients:

- 2 fennel bulbs, sliced
- 2 tablespoons olive oil
- 4 garlic cloves, chopped
- 2 tablespoons balsamic vinegar
- 2 and ½ cups baby spinach
- ½ teaspoon nutmeg, ground
- ¼ cup veggie stock

Directions:

In your instant pot, combine the fennel with the spinach and the rest of the ingredients, put the lid on and cook on High for 10 minutes. Release the pressure naturally for 10 minutes, divide the mix between plates and serve.

Nutrition: calories 104, fat 7.4, fiber 3.6, carbs 6.4, protein 1.7

Dill Cherry Tomatoes

Preparation time: 10 minutes | Cooking time: 12 minutes | Servings: 4

Ingredients:

- 4 garlic cloves, minced
- A pinch of salt and black pepper
- 2 pounds cherry tomatoes, halved
- 2 tablespoons olive oil
- 1 tablespoon dill, chopped
- ½ cups chicken stock
- ¼ cup basil, chopped

Directions:

Set your instant pot on sauté mode, add the oil, heat it up, add the garlic and sauté for 2 minutes. Add the rest of the ingredients, put the lid on and cook on High for 10 minutes. Release the pressure naturally for 10 minutes, divide the mix between plates and serve.

Nutrition: calories 109, fat 7.6, fiber 2.9, carbs 6.8, protein 2.5

Tomatoes and Cauliflower Mix

Preparation time: 10 minutes | Cooking time: 12 minutes | Servings: 4

Ingredients:

- ½ cup scallions, chopped
- 1 tablespoon avocado oil
- 1 pound cauliflower florets
- ½ cup chicken stock
- 2 cups cherry tomatoes, halved
- 1 tablespoon chives, chopped
- 2 tablespoons parsley, chopped

Directions:

Set your instant pot on Sauté mode, add the oil, heat it up, add the scallions and sauté for 2 minutes. Add the rest of the ingredients, put the lid on and cook on High for 10 minutes. Release the pressure naturally for 10 minutes, divide the mix between plates and serve as a side dish.

Nutrition: calories 55, fat 1.6, fiber 0.4, carbs 1.5, protein 3.5

Green Beans and Herbs
Preparation time: 10 minutes | Cooking time: 12 minutes | Servings: 4

Ingredients:
- 2 tablespoons avocado oil
- ½ teaspoon chili powder
- 1 pound green beans, trimmed and halved
- 1 and ½ cups chicken stock
- 1 tablespoon rosemary, chopped
- 1 tablespoon basil, chopped
- 1 tablespoon dill, chopped
- A pinch of salt and black pepper
- ½ cup almonds, chopped

Directions:
In your instant pot, combine the green beans with the chili and the rest of the ingredients. put the lid on and cook on High for 12 minutes. Release the pressure naturally for 10 minutes, divide the mix between plates and serve as a side dish.

Nutrition: calories 119, fat 7.2, fiber 3.4, carbs 5.3, protein 4.9

Cauliflower Rice and Olives
Preparation time: 10 minutes | Cooking time: 15 minutes | Servings: 4

Ingredients:
- 1 cup cauliflower rice
- 1 and ½ cup chicken stock
- 1 cup black olives, pitted and sliced
- 1 tablespoon chives, chopped
- A pinch of salt and black pepper
- ½ cup cilantro, chopped

Directions:
In your instant pot, mix the cauliflower rice with the rest of the ingredients, put the lid on and cook on High for 15 minutes. Release the pressure naturally for 10 minutes, divide the mix between plates and serve.

Nutrition: calories 40, fat 3.6, fiber 1.2, carbs 2.2, protein 0.3

Rosemary Cauliflower

Preparation time: 10 minutes | Cooking time: 12 minutes | Servings: 4

Ingredients:

- 1 pound cauliflower florets
- 1 cup chicken stock
- 2 garlic cloves, minced
- A pinch of salt and black pepper
- 1 tablespoon rosemary, chopped
- 1 teaspoon hot chili sauce

Directions:

In your instant pot, combine the cauliflower with the stock and the rest of the ingredients, put the lid on and cook on High for 12 minutes. Release the pressure naturally for 10 minutes, divide the mix between plates and serve.

Nutrition: calories 36, fat 2.4, fiber 1.5, carbs 2.3, protein 3.6

Lemon Artichokes

Preparation time: 10 minutes | Cooking time: 12 minutes | Servings: 4

Ingredients:

- 4 artichokes, trimmed
- 1 tablespoon olive oil
- 1 tablespoon lemon juice
- 1 tablespoon chives, chopped
- 1 tablespoon sweet paprika
- 1 tablespoon parsley, chopped
- 2 cups water

Directions:

In a bowl, mix the artichokes with the oil and the other ingredients except the water and toss. Put the water in your instant pot, add the steamer basket, put the artichokes inside, put the lid on and cook on High for 12 minutes. Release the pressure naturally for 10 minutes, divide the artichokes between plates and serve.

Nutrition: calories 113, fat 4, fiber 2.4, carbs 3.5, protein 5.6

Celery and Broccoli Mix

Preparation time: 10 minutes | Cooking time: 12 minutes | Servings: 4

Ingredients:

- 2 garlic cloves, minced
- 1 tablespoon olive oil
- 1 and ½ cups broccoli florets
- 1 celery stalk, chopped
- ½ cups veggie stock
- A pinch of salt and black pepper
- 2 tablespoons lime juice

Directions:

Set your instant pot on sauté mode, add the oil, heat it up, add the garlic and celery and cook for 2 minutes. Add the rest of the ingredients, put the lid on and cook on High for 10 minutes. Release the pressure naturally for 10 minutes, divide the mix between plates and serve.

Nutrition: calories 33, fat 3.5, fiber 0.1, carbs 0.7, protein 0.1

Zucchini Mix

Preparation time: 10 minutes | Cooking time: 20 minutes | Servings: 4

Ingredients:

- ½ cup veggie stock
- 3 zucchinis, sliced
- A pinch of salt and black pepper
- 1 tablespoon dill, chopped
- ½ teaspoon nutmeg, grated
- 2 tablespoons sweet paprika

Directions:

In your instant pot, mix the zucchinis with the rest of the ingredients, put the lid on and cook on Low for 20 minutes. Release the pressure naturally for 10 minutes, divide the mix between plates and serve.

Nutrition: calories 40, fat 2.3, fiber 1.5, carbs 1.9, protein 2.5

Dill Fennel Mix

Preparation time: 10 minutes | Cooking time: 10 minutes | Servings: 4

Ingredients:

- 2 fennel bulbs, sliced
- ¼ cup chicken stock
- A pinch of salt and black pepper
- 1 tablespoon dill, chopped
- 1 tablespoon parsley, chopped

Directions:

In your instant pot, mix the fennel with the stock and the rest of the ingredients, put the lid on and cook on High for 10 minutes. Release the pressure naturally for 10 minutes, divide the mix between plates and serve.

Nutrition: calories 39, fat 3.2, fiber 1, carbs 2.9, protein 1.7

Mushrooms and Endives Mix

Preparation time: 10 minutes | Cooking time: 15 minutes | Servings: 4

Ingredients:

- 1 pound white mushrooms, sliced
- 2 spring onions, chopped
- 1 garlic clove, minced
- 2 endives, trimmed and halved
- 1 tablespoon balsamic vinegar
- 1 tablespoon chives, chopped
- 1 cup chicken stock

Directions:

In your instant pot, mix the mushrooms with the rest of the ingredients, put the lid on and cook on High for 15 minutes. Release the pressure naturally for 10 minutes, divide the mix between plates and serve.

Nutrition: calories 31, fat 3.1, fiber 1.3, carbs 2.3, protein 3.9

Walnuts Green Beans and Avocado

Preparation time: 10 minutes | Cooking time: 15 minutes | Servings: 6

Ingredients:

- 2 cups green beans, halved
- ½ cup chicken stock
- ½ cup walnuts, chopped
- 1 avocado, peeled, pitted and cubed
- ¼ teaspoon sweet paprika
- A pinch of salt and black pepper
- 2 teaspoons balsamic vinegar

Directions:

In your instant pot, mix the green beans with the stock and the rest of the ingredients, put the lid on and cook on High for 15 minutes. Release the pressure naturally for 10 minutes, divide the mix between plates and serve.

Nutrition: calories 146, fat 12.8, fiber 2.5, carbs 6.7, protein 3.9

Thyme Brussels Sprouts

Preparation time: 10 minutes | Cooking time: 12 minutes | Servings: 4

Ingredients:

- 2 and ½ pounds Brussels sprouts, halved
- 2 tablespoons olive oil
- A pinch of salt and black pepper
- 2 shallots, chopped
- ½ cups beef stock
- 1 tablespoon thyme, chopped

Directions:

Set your instant pot on Sauté mode, add the oil, heat it up, add the shallots and sauté for 2 minutes. Add the rest of the ingredients, put the lid on and cook on High or 10 minutes. Release the pressure naturally for 10 minutes, divide the mix between plates and serve as a side dish.

Nutrition: calories 64, fat 7.1, fiber 0.3, carbs 0.5, protein 0.4

Chives Broccoli Mash

Preparation time: 10 minutes | Cooking time: 12 minutes | Servings: 4

Ingredients:

- 1 broccoli, florets separated
- A pinch of salt and black pepper
- ½ teaspoon turmeric powder
- ½ cup chicken stock
- 1 tablespoon ghee, melted
- 1 tablespoon chives, chopped

Directions:

In your instant pot, mix the broccoli with the rest of the ingredients except the ghee and the chives, put the lid on and cook on High for 12 minutes. Release the pressure naturally for 10 minutes, drain the broccoli, transfer it to a blender, add the ghee, pulse well, divide between plates, sprinkle the chives on top and serve.

Nutrition: calories 31, fat 3.3, fiber 0.1, carbs 0.3, protein 0.1

Creamy Endives

Preparation time: 10 minutes | Cooking time: 10 minutes | Servings: 4

Ingredients:

- 4 endives, trimmed and halved
- ½ cup chicken stock
- ¼ cup coconut cream
- 1 tablespoon dill, chopped
- 1 tablespoon smoked paprika

Directions:

In your instant pot, mix the endives with the rest of the ingredients, put the lid on and cook on High for 10 minutes. Release the pressure naturally for 10 minutes, divide the mix between plates and serve as a side dish.

Nutrition: calories 43, fat 3.9, fiber 1.1, carbs 2.3, protein 0.9

Spinach and Kale Mix

Preparation time: 5 minutes | Cooking time: 10 minutes | Servings: 4

Ingredients:

- 1 and ½ pounds baby spinach
- ½ pound kale, torn
- 1 tablespoon ghee, melted
- A pinch of salt and black pepper
- 1 cup veggie stock
- 1 teaspoon nutmeg, ground
- 1 tablespoon chives, chopped

Directions:

In your instant pot, mix the spinach with the kale and the rest of the ingredients, toss, put the lid on and cook on High for 10 minutes. Release the pressure fast for 5 minutes, divide the mix between plates and serve.

Nutrition: calories 59, fat 3.4, fiber 1, carbs 2.4, protein 1.8

Thyme Tomatoes

Preparation time: 10 minutes | Cooking time: 10 minutes | Servings: 4

Ingredients:

- ½ cup veggie stock
- 1 pound cherry tomatoes, halved
- 1 tablespoon thyme, chopped
- A pinch of salt and black pepper
- 1 teaspoon chili powder
- 1 shallot, chopped
- 1 tablespoon olive oil

Directions:

Set the instant pot on Sauté mode, add the oil, heat it up, add the shallot and sauté for 2 minutes. Add the tomatoes and the rest of the ingredients, put the lid on and cook on High for 8 minutes. Release the pressure naturally for 10 minutes, divide the mix between plates and serve.

Nutrition: calories 54, fat 3.9, fiber 1.8, carbs 2.4, protein 1.1

Lemon Brussels Sprouts and Tomatoes

Preparation time: 10 minutes | Cooking time: 15 minutes | Servings: 4

Ingredients:

- 1 pound Brussels sprouts, trimmed and halved
- ½ pound cherry tomatoes, halved
- 1 tablespoon lemon juice
- 1 tablespoon lemon zest, grated
- ¼ cup veggie stock
- 1 tablespoon rosemary, chopped
- A pinch of salt and black pepper

Directions:

In your instant pot, mix the Brussels sprouts with the tomatoes and the remaining ingredients, put the lid on and cook on High for 15 minutes. Release the pressure naturally for 10 minutes, divide the mix between plates and serve as a side dish.

Nutrition: calories 64, fat 2.7, fiber 1.5, carbs 2, protein 4.5

Creamy Fennel

Preparation time: 5 minutes | Cooking time: 8 minutes | Servings: 4

Ingredients:

- 2 big fennel bulbs, sliced
- 2 tablespoons avocado oil
- 2 spring onions, chopped
- 2 shallots, minced
- 1 garlic clove, minced
- 1 and ½ cups coconut cream
- ¼ teaspoon nutmeg, ground
- A pinch of salt and black pepper

Directions:

Set your instant pot on Sauté mode, add the oil, heat it up, add spring onions, shallots and the garlic and sauté for 2 minutes. Add the fennel and the rest of the ingredients, toss, put the lid on and cook on High for 6 minutes. Release the pressure fast for 5 minutes, divide the mix between plates and serve as a side dish.

Nutrition: calories 58, fat 3.2, fiber 1, carbs 2.7, protein 0.3

Saffron Bell Peppers

Preparation time: 10 minutes | Cooking time: 10 minutes | Servings: 4

Ingredients:

- 2 yellow bell peppers, cut into strips
- 2 red bell peppers, thinly sliced
- 3 garlic cloves, minced
- 1 shallots, chopped
- A pinch of salt and black pepper
- 1 teaspoon saffron powder
- ¼ cup chicken stock
- 1 tablespoon cilantro, chopped

Directions:

In your instant pot, mix the peppers with the garlic and the rest of the ingredients, put the lid on and cook on High for 10 minutes. Release the pressure naturally for 10 minutes, divide the mix between plates and serve.

Nutrition: calories 64, fat 2.4, fiber 1.7, carbs 1.9, protein 1.4

Cabbage and Peppers

Preparation time: 10 minutes | Cooking time: 15 minutes | Servings: 4

Ingredients:

- 2 red bell peppers, cut into strips
- 1 green cabbage head, shredded
- ½ cup chicken stock
- 1 tablespoon avocado oil
- 1 tablespoon sweet paprika
- A pinch of salt and black pepper
- 2 garlic cloves, minced
- 1 teaspoon lime zest, grated
- 1 teaspoon lime juice
- 1 tablespoon dill, chopped

Directions:

Set the instant pot on Sauté mode, add the oil, heat it up, add the garlic, lime zest and lime juice and sauté for 2 minutes. Add the peppers and the rest of the ingredients, put the lid on and cook on High for 12 minutes. Release the pressure naturally for 10 minutes, divide the mix between plates and serve.

Nutrition: calories 79, fat 2.6, fiber 0.4, carbs 1.4, protein 3.5

Green Beans and Kale

Preparation time: 10 minutes | Cooking time: 8 minutes | Servings: 4

Ingredients:

- 2 cups kale, torn
- 1 tablespoon avocado oil
- 1 garlic clove, minced
- 1 pound green beans, trimmed
- 1 tablespoon chives, chopped
- 1 tablespoon oregano, chopped
- ¼ cup chicken stock
- 1 teaspoon chili powder

Directions:

Set your instant pot on Sauté mode, add the oil, heat it up, add the garlic and cook for 1 minute. Add the rest of the ingredients, put the lid on and cook on High for 7 minutes. Release the pressure naturally for 10 minutes, divide the mix between plates and serve.

Nutrition: calories 64, fat 1.9, fiber 0.5, carbs 1.4, protein 3.4

Zucchinis and Bok Choy

Preparation time: 10 minutes | Cooking time: 10 minutes | Servings: 4

Ingredients:

- 2 bunches bok choy
- 3 zucchinis, sliced
- ¼ cup veggie stock
- 2 garlic cloves, minced
- 1 teaspoon ginger, grated
- 1 tablespoon avocado oil
- 1 tablespoon smoked paprika
- A pinch of salt and black pepper
- 1 tablespoon dill, chopped

Directions:

Set the instant pot on Sauté mode, add the oil, heat it up, add the ginger and the garlic and sauté for 2 minutes. Add the bok choy and the rest of the ingredients, put the lid on and cook on High for 8 minutes. Release the pressure naturally for 10 minutes, divide everything between plates and serve as a side dish.

Nutrition: calories 49, fat 1, fiber 0.2, carbs 0.3, protein 2.4

Red Cabbage and Artichokes

Preparation time: 10 minutes | Cooking time: 15 minutes | Servings: 4

Ingredients:

- 4 garlic cloves, minced
- ½ cup spring onions, chopped
- 1 tablespoon avocado oil
- 1 red cabbage head, shredded
- ¼ cup veggie stock
- 1 cup canned artichokes hearts, drained and chopped
- 1 tablespoon balsamic vinegar
- 1 tablespoon dill, chopped

Directions:

Set your instant pot on Sauté mode, add the oil, heat it up, add the garlic and the onions and sauté for 2 minutes. Add the rest of the ingredients, put the lid on and cook on High for 13 minutes. Release the pressure naturally for 10 minutes, divide the mix between plates and serve.

Nutrition: calories 69, fat 2.3, fiber 1.9, carbs 2, protein 2.9

Balsamic Artichokes and Capers

Preparation time: 10 minutes | Cooking time: 15 minutes | Servings: 4

Ingredients:

- 4 artichokes, trimmed
- 1 cup water
- 2 tablespoons balsamic vinegar
- 2 tablespoons capers, drained and chopped
- 1 tablespoon chives, chopped
- A pinch of salt and black pepper
- 1 tablespoon avocado oil

Directions:

In a bowl, mix the artichokes with the rest of the ingredients except the water and the capers and toss. Put the water in the instant pot, add the steamer basket, put the artichokes inside, put the lid on and cook on High for 15 minutes. Release the pressure naturally for 10 minutes, divide the artichokes between plates, sprinkle the capers on top and serve.

Nutrition: calories 84, fat 1.9, fiber 1, carbs 1.5, protein 5.5

Bell Peppers and Olives

Preparation time: 10 minutes | Cooking time: 12 minutes | Servings: 4

Ingredients:

- 1 and ½ pounds mixed bell peppers, cut into strips
- 2 teaspoons lemon zest, grated
- 2 tablespoons lemon juice
- 2 scallions, chopped
- 1 cup black olives, pitted and halved
- ¼ cup veggie stock

Directions:

In your instant pot, mix the peppers with the lemon zest and the rest of the ingredients, put the lid on and cook on High for 12 minutes. Release the pressure naturally for 10 minutes, divide the mix between plates and serve.

Nutrition: calories 44, fat 3.7, fiber 1.4, carbs 3, protein 0.5

Tomatoes and Olives

Preparation time: 10 minutes | Cooking time: 15 minutes | Servings: 4

Ingredients:

- 1 pound cherry tomatoes, halved
- 1 cup kalamata olives, pitted and halved
- 2 tablespoons goat cheese, crumbled
- 1 tablespoon balsamic vinegar
- ¼ cup veggie stock
- 1 tablespoon chives, chopped
- A pinch of salt and black pepper

Directions:

In your instant pot, mix the tomatoes with the olives and the rest of the ingredients except the cheese and the stock, put the lid on and cook on High for 15 minutes. Release the pressure naturally for 10 minutes, divide the mix between plates, sprinkle the cheese and the chives on top and serve.

Nutrition: calories 60, fat 3.8, fiber 2.1, carbs 3.5, protein 1.3

Balsamic Eggplant Mix
Preparation time: 10 minutes | Cooking time: 12 minutes | Servings: 4
Ingredients:

- 2 eggplants, sliced
- ¼ cup veggie stock
- 1 tablespoon olive oil
- 6 garlic cloves, minced
- 1 tablespoon balsamic vinegar
- 1 tablespoon chives, chopped
- A pinch of salt and black pepper

Directions:

Set the instant pot on Sauté mode, add the oil, heat it up, add the garlic and sauté for 2 minutes. Add the eggplants and the rest of the ingredients, put the lid on and cook on High for 10 minutes. Release the pressure naturally for 10 minutes, divide the mix between plates and serve.

Nutrition: calories 106, fat 4, fiber 1.9, carbs 2.7, protein 3

Buttery Eggplants
Preparation time: 5 minutes | Cooking time: 12 minutes | Servings: 4
Ingredients:

- 1 pound eggplants, sliced
- A pinch of salt and black pepper
- 2 shallots, chopped
- 1 cup chicken stock
- 1 tablespoon ghee, melted
- 2 tablespoons parsley, chopped

Directions:

Set your instant pot on Sauté mode, add the ghee, heat it up, add the shallots and cook for 2 minutes. Add the eggplants and the rest of the ingredients, put the lid on and cook on High for 10 minutes. Release the pressure fast for 5 minutes, divide the mix between plates and serve.

Nutrition: calories 60, fat 3.5, fiber 1.8, carbs 3, protein 1.4

Bacon Artichokes
Preparation time: 10 minutes | Cooking time: 12 minutes | Servings: 4
Ingredients:

- 1 cup bacon, chopped
- 1 pound canned artichokes hearts, drained
- ¼ teaspoon nutmeg, ground
- A pinch of salt and black pepper
- 1 cup coconut milk
- 2 tablespoons parsley, chopped

Directions:

In your instant pot, combine the artichokes with the rest of the ingredients, put the lid on and cook on High for 12 minutes. Release the pressure naturally for 10 minutes, divide the mix between plates and serve as a side dish.

Nutrition: calories 140, fat 14.2, fiber 1.4, carbs 3.5, protein 1.4

Cabbage and Tomatoes
Preparation time: 10 minutes | Cooking time: 15 minutes | Servings: 4

Ingredients:
- 1 green cabbage, shredded
- 1 pound cherry tomatoes, halved
- 1 shallot, chopped
- 1 tablespoon olive oil
- ¼ cup balsamic vinegar
- ¼ cup veggie stock
- A pinch of cayenne pepper
- 1 tablespoon dill, chopped

Directions:
Set your instant pot on Sauté mode, add the oil, heat it up, add the shallot and sauté for 2 minutes. Add the cabbage and the rest of the ingredients, put the lid on and cook on High for 13 minutes. Release the pressure naturally for 10 minutes, divide the mix between plates and serve.

Nutrition: calories 56, fat 3.8, fiber 1.5, carbs 3, protein 1.2

Balsamic Collard Greens
Preparation time: 10 minutes | Cooking time: 15 minutes | Servings: 4

Ingredients:
- 1 bunch collard greens, trimmed
- 2 tablespoons avocado oil
- ½ cup chicken stock
- 2 tablespoons balsamic vinegar
- 3 garlic cloves, minced
- A pinch of salt and black pepper
- 1 tablespoon chives, chopped

Directions:
Set the instant pot on Sauté mode, add the oil, heat it up, add the garlic and cook for 2 minutes. Add the collard greens and the rest of the ingredients, put the lid on and cook on High for 13 minutes. Release the pressure naturally for 10 minutes, divide everything between plates and serve as a side dish.

Nutrition: calories 73, fat 2.1, fiber 0.3, carbs 1.4, protein 0.3

Cilantro Cauliflower Rice Mix

Preparation time: 10 minutes | Cooking time: 15 minutes | Servings: 4

Ingredients:

- 1 shallot, chopped
- 1 teaspoon garlic, minced
- 1 tablespoon avocado oil
- 1 and ½ cups cauliflower rice
- 1 and ½ cups chicken stock
- A pinch of salt and black pepper
- 2 tablespoons chives, chopped

Directions:

Set your instant pot on Sauté mode, add the oil, heat it up, add the shallot and the garlic and sauté for 2 minutes. Add the rest of the ingredients except the chives, put the lid on and cook on High for 13 minutes. Release the pressure naturally for 10 minutes, divide the mix between plates and serve as a side dish.

Nutrition: calories 55, fat 2.3, fiber 0.2, carbs 0.3, protein 0.1

Leeks Sauté

Preparation time: 10 minutes | Cooking time: 10 minutes | Servings: 4

Ingredients:

- 2 scallions, chopped
- 4 leeks, sliced
- A pinch of salt and black pepper
- 1 teaspoon chili powder
- ¼ cup chicken stock
- 2 tablespoons parsley, chopped
- 1 tablespoon lemon zest, grated

Directions:

In your instant pot, combine the leeks with the rest of the ingredients, put the lid on and cook on High for 10 minutes. Release the pressure naturally for 10 minutes, divide the mix between plates and serve.

Nutrition: calories 61, fat 2.5, fiber 1.1, carbs 2.1, protein 1.7

Eggplant and Zucchini Mix

Preparation time: 10 minutes | Cooking time: 12 minutes | Servings: 4

Ingredients:

- 2 eggplants, cubed
- 2 zucchinis, roughly cubed
- 1 tablespoon chives, chopped
- ¼ cup chicken stock
- 1 teaspoon chili powder
- 1 tablespoon oregano, chopped
- A pinch of salt and black pepper
- 2 tablespoons parsley, chopped

Directions:

In your instant pot, combine the eggplants with the zucchinis and the rest of the ingredients, put the lid on and cook on High for 12 minutes. Release the pressure naturally for 10 minutes, divide the mix between plates and serve.

Nutrition: calories 91, fat 1, fiber 0.2, carbs 0.3, protein 4.2

Chili Cauliflower Rice

Preparation time: 10 minutes | Cooking time: 20 minutes | Servings: 4

Ingredients:

- A pinch of salt and black pepper
- ½ teaspoon cayenne pepper
- 1 teaspoon chili powder
- 2 tablespoons green onions, chopped
- 1 cup chicken stock
- 2 cups cauliflower rice

Directions:

In your instant pot, mix the cauliflower rice with the stock and the rest of the ingredients, put the lid on and cook on Low for 20 minutes. Release the pressure naturally for 10 minutes, divide the mix between plates and serve.

Nutrition: calories 52, fat 1.5, fiber 0.2, carbs 0.3, protein 0.7

Sage Eggplants and Green Beans

Preparation time: 10 minutes | Cooking time: 15 minutes | Servings: 4

Ingredients:

- 2 cups green beans, trimmed and halved
- 1 cup chicken stock
- 2 garlic cloves, minced
- 2 eggplants, roughly cubed
- 2 tablespoon olive oil
- 2 tablespoons sage, chopped
- 2 tablespoons parmesan, grated

Directions:

Set your instant pot on Sauté mode, add the oil, heat it up, add the garlic and cook for 2 minutes. Add the green beans and the rest of the ingredients except the parmesan, put the lid on and cook on High for 13 minutes. Release the pressure naturally for 10 minutes, divide the mix between plates, sprinkle the parmesan on top and serve.

Nutrition: calories 152, fat 7.8, fiber 2.1, carbs 4.3, protein 4.1

Nutmeg Zucchini Rice

Preparation time: 10 minutes | Cooking time: 15 minutes | Servings: 4

Ingredients:

- 2 tablespoons avocado oil
- 1 shallot, chopped
- 2 garlic cloves, minced
- 2 cups cauliflower rice
- 1 and ½ cups chicken stock
- 1 big zucchini, grated
- ½ teaspoon allspice, ground
- 1 tablespoon parsley, chopped

Directions:

Set your instant pot on Sauté mode, add the oil, heat it up, add the shallot and the garlic and sauté for 2 minutes. Add the rest of the ingredients, toss, put the lid on and cook on High for 13 minutes. Release the pressure naturally for 10 minutes, divide the mix between plates and serve as a side dish.

Nutrition: calories 62, fat 1.7, fiber 1, carbs 1.4, protein 1.2

Spiced Zucchinis

Preparation time: 5 minutes | Cooking time: 15 minutes | Servings: 4

Ingredients:

- 1 teaspoon ginger, grated
- 3 garlic cloves, minced
- 2 zucchinis, sliced
- 1 tablespoon olive oil
- 1 tablespoon cumin, ground
- 1 teaspoon cardamom, ground
- 1 teaspoon sweet paprika
- A pinch of salt and black pepper

Directions:

Set the instant pot on sauté mode, add the oil, heat it up, add the garlic and the ginger and sauté for 2 minutes. Add the remaining ingredients, put the lid on and cook on High for 13 minutes. Release the pressure fast for 5 minutes, divide the mix between plates and serve.

Nutrition: calories 59, fat 4.2, fiber 1.5, carbs 2.4, protein 1.9

Leeks and Cabbage

Preparation time: 10 minutes | Cooking time: 10 minutes | Servings: 4

Ingredients:

- 2 garlic cloves, minced
- 3 leeks, sliced
- 1 green cabbage, shredded
- A pinch of salt and black pepper
- ½ teaspoon rosemary, dried
- ½ teaspoon thyme dried
- ½ cup chicken stock

Directions:

In your instant pot, mix the leeks with the cabbage and the rest of the ingredients, put the lid on and cook on High for 10 minutes. Release the pressure naturally for 10 minutes, divide the mix between plates and serve as a side dish.

Nutrition: calories 55, fat 1.6, fiber 0.7, carbs 1.1, protein 1.2

Cranberries Cauliflower Rice

Preparation time: 10 minutes | Cooking time: 15 minutes | Servings: 4

Ingredients:

- 2 tablespoons avocado oil
- 2 shallots, chopped
- ½ cup cranberries
- 1 and ½ cups cauliflower rice
- 1 cup veggie stock
- A pinch of salt and black pepper
- ½ cup cilantro, chopped

Directions:

Set your instant pot on Sauté mode, add the oil, heat it up, add the shallots and sauté for 2 minutes Add the rest of the ingredients, stir, put the lid on and cook on High for 13 minutes. Release the pressure naturally for 10 minutes, divide the mix between plates and serve as a side dish.

Nutrition: calories 34, fat 2, fiber 0.2, carbs 1.7, protein 1

Mint Zucchinis

Preparation time: 10 minutes | Cooking time: 12 minutes | Servings: 4

Ingredients:

- 1 tablespoon balsamic vinegar
- 2 zucchinis, sliced
- 1 teaspoon lime juice
- A pinch of salt and black pepper
- ¼ cup chicken stock
- 1 tablespoon olive oil
- ½ cup green onions, chopped
- 2 tablespoons mint, chopped

Directions:

Set the instant pot on Sauté mode, add the oil, heat it up, add the onions and sauté for 2 minutes. Add the rest of the ingredients, put the lid on and cook on High for 10 minutes. Release the pressure naturally for 10 minutes, divide the mix between plates and serve.

Nutrition: calories 52, fat 3.8, fiber 1.6, carbs 2.3, protein 1.6

Ketogenic Instant Pot Snack and Appetizer Recipes

Lemon Zucchini and Eggplant Spread
Preparation time: 10 minutes | Cooking time: 15 minutes | Servings: 4

Ingredients:

- 2 and ½ teaspoons lemon zest, grated
- 3 tablespoons lemon juice
- 2 zucchinis, chopped
- 2 eggplants, chopped
- 1 tablespoon olive oil
- ½ cup veggie stock
- 2 tablespoons dill, chopped

Directions:

In your instant pot, the zucchinis with the eggplants and the rest of the ingredients, except the dill, put the lid on and cook on High for 15 minutes. Release the pressure naturally for 10 minutes, blend the mix with an immersion blender, divide into bowls, sprinkle the dill on top and serve.

Nutrition: calories 121, fat 4.3, fiber 1, carbs 1.4, protein 4.3

Oregano Green Beans Salsa
Preparation time: 10 minutes | Cooking time: 10 minutes | Servings: 4

Ingredients:

- 1 pound green beans, trimmed and halved
- ¼ cup veggie stock
- 1 tablespoon olive oil
- 2 garlic cloves, minced
- A pinch of salt and black pepper
- 2 tomatoes, cubed
- 2 cucumbers, cubed
- 1 avocado, peeled, pitted and cubed
- 2 tablespoons balsamic vinegar
- 1 tablespoon oregano, chopped

Directions:

In your instant pot mix the green beans with the stock, garlic, salt and pepper, put the lid on and cook on High for 10 minutes. Release the pressure naturally for 10 minutes, transfer the green beans to a bowl, add the rest of the ingredients, toss, divide the salsa into cups and serve.

Nutrition: calories 209, fat 11.2, fiber 3, carbs 4.4, protein 4.8

Basil Zucchini and Capers Dip

Preparation time: 10 minutes | *Cooking time:* 10 minutes | *Servings:* 4

Ingredients:

- 1 shallot, chopped
- 1 and ½ pounds zucchinis, chopped
- 1 tablespoon olive oil
- 2 garlic cloves, minced
- A pinch of salt and black pepper
- 1 tablespoon capers, drained and chopped
- ¼ cup veggie stock
- 1 bunch basil, chopped

Directions:

Set your instant pot on Sauté mode, add the oil, heat it up, add the shallot and the garlic, stir and sauté for 2 minutes. Add the zucchinis and the rest of the ingredients, put the lid on and cook on High for 8 minutes. Release the pressure naturally for 10 minutes, blend everything using an immersion blender, divide into bowls and serve.

Nutrition: calories 75, fat 2.5, fiber 0.1, carbs 0.6, protein 1.2

Lime Spinach and Leeks Dip

Preparation time: 10 minutes | *Cooking time:* 20 minutes | *Servings:* 4

Ingredients:

- 1 shallot, chopped
- 2 tablespoons avocado oil
- 2 leeks, chopped
- 2 garlic cloves, minced
- 4 cups spinach, torn
- ¼ cup veggie stock
- ¼ cup lime juice
- 1 bunch basil, chopped
- A pinch of salt and black pepper

Directions:

Set your instant pot on Sauté mode, add the oil, heat it up, add the shallot, leeks and garlic and sauté for 5 minutes. Add the rest of the ingredients, put the lid on and cook on High for 15 minutes. Release the pressure naturally for 10 minutes, blend the mix using an immersion blender, transfer to bowls and serve as a snack.

Nutrition: calories 56, fat 1.8, fiber 0.5, carbs 1.6, protein 1.7

Chili Tomato and Zucchini Dip

Preparation time: 10 minutes | Cooking time: 15 minutes | Servings: 4

Ingredients:

- 2 cups tomatoes, cubed
- 2 cups zucchinis, cubed
- 1 tablespoon hot paprika
- 2 red chilies, chopped
- ¼ cup veggie stock
- 1 tablespoon basil, chopped
- A pinch of salt and black pepper
- 2 scallions, chopped
- 1 tablespoon olive oil

Directions:

Set the instant pot on Sauté mode, add the oil, heat it up, add the chilies and the scallions and sauté for 2 minutes. Add the tomatoes and the rest of the ingredients except the basil, put the lid on and cook on High for 12 minutes. Release the pressure naturally for 10 minutes, blend the mix with an immersion blender, divide into bowls, sprinkle the basil on top and serve.

Nutrition: calories 58, fat 3.5, fiber 1.9, carbs 2.3, protein 1.6

Parmesan Mushroom Spread

Preparation time: 10 minutes | Cooking time: 20 minutes | Servings: 4

Ingredients:

- 1 shallot chopped
- 2 tablespoons olive oil
- 1 tablespoon rosemary, chopped
- A pinch of salt and black pepper
- 3 garlic cloves, minced
- 1 cup chicken stock
- 2 pounds white mushrooms, sliced
- ½ cup parmesan, grated
- ½ cup coconut cream
- 1 tablespoons parsley, chopped

Directions:

Set your instant pot on Sauté mode, add the oil, heat it up, add the shallot and garlic and sauté for 2 minutes. Add the mushrooms and sauté for 5 minutes. Add the rest of the ingredients, put the lid on and cook on High for 15 minutes. Release the pressure naturally, divide the mix into bowls and serve as a party spread.

Nutrition: calories 187, fat 12.4, fiber 2.1, carbs 4.5, protein 8.2

Broccoli Dip

Preparation time: 10 minutes | Cooking time: 15 minutes | Servings: 6

Ingredients:
- 2 tablespoons avocado oil
- 8 garlic cloves, minced
- 2 cups veggie stock
- 6 cups broccoli florets
- 1 cup Greek yogurt
- 1 tablespoon dill, chopped
- A pinch of salt and black pepper
- ½ cup coconut cream

Directions:

Set your instant pot on Sauté mode, add the oil, heat it up, add the garlic and cook for 2 minutes. Add the rest of the ingredients except the dill and the yogurt, put the lid on and cook on High for 13 minutes. Release the pressure naturally for 10 minutes, add the yogurt, blend the mix with an immersion blender, divide into bowls, sprinkle the dill on top and serve.

Nutrition: calories 136, fat 8.6, fiber 4.8, carbs 5.6, protein 5.1

Ginger Cauliflower Spread

Preparation time: 10 minutes | Cooking time: 15 minutes | Servings: 4

Ingredients:
- 1 shallot, chopped
- 1 tablespoon avocado oil
- 2 tablespoons ginger, minced
- 1 pound cauliflower florets
- ¼ cup chicken stock
- 2 red hot chilies, chopped
- 1 and ¼ tablespoon balsamic vinegar

Directions:

Set your instant pot on Sauté mode, add the oil, heat it up, add the ginger and the shallot and sauté for 2 minutes. Add the rest of the ingredients, put the lid on and cook on High for 13 minutes. Release the pressure naturally for 10 minutes, blend the mix a bit with an immersion blender, divide into bowls and serve as a party spread.

Nutrition: calories 45, fat 2.5, fiber 1.3, carbs 2, protein 2.6

Radish Salsa

Preparation time: 10 minutes | Cooking time: 15 minutes | Servings: 4

Ingredients:

- 2 cups red radishes, sliced
- 1 shallot, chopped
- 2 spring onions, chopped
- 2 tomatoes, cubed
- 1 avocado, peeled and cubed
- 1 tablespoon olive oil
- ¼ cup chicken stock
- A pinch of salt and black pepper
- 1 tablespoon oregano, chopped
- 1 tablespoon chives, chopped

Directions:

In your instant pot, combine the radishes with the stock, oregano, salt and pepper, put the lid on and cook on Low for 15 minutes. Release the pressure naturally for 10 minutes, transfer the radishes to a bowl, add the rest of the ingredients, toss, divide into small cups and serve as an appetizer.

Nutrition: calories 160, fat 13.7, fiber 5.5, carbs 10.1, protein 2.2

Mustard Greens Dip

Preparation time: 5 minutes | Cooking time: 14 minutes | Servings: 4

Ingredients:

- 6 ounces mustard greens, chopped
- 1 tablespoon olive oil
- 1 tablespoon basil, chopped
- 1 garlic clove, minced
- ¼ cup veggie stock
- 1 tablespoon balsamic vinegar
- 2 tablespoon coconut cream
- A pinch of salt and black pepper

Directions:

Set your instant pot on Sauté mode, add the oil, heat it up, add the garlic and cook for 1 minute Add the rest of the ingredients, put the lid on and cook on High for 13 minutes. Release the pressure fast for 5 minutes, blend the mix with an immersion blender, divide into bowls and serve.

Nutrition: calories 60, fat 5.4, fiber 1.6, carbs 2.8, protein 1.4

Spinach and Artichokes Spread

Preparation time: 10 minutes | Cooking time: 15 minutes | Servings: 6

Ingredients:

- 14 ounces canned artichoke hearts, drained
- 8 ounces mozzarella cheese, shredded
- 1 pound spinach, torn
- 1 teaspoon garlic powder
- ½ cup chicken stock
- ½ cup coconut cream
- A pinch of salt and black pepper

Directions:

In your instant pot, mix the artichokes with the rest of the ingredients, put the lid on and cook on High for 15 minutes. Release the pressure naturally for 10 minutes, blend the mix using an immersion blender, stir well, transfer to a bowl and serve as a snack.

Nutrition: calories 204, fat 11.5, fiber 3.1, carbs 4.2, protein 5.9

Artichokes and Salmon Bowls

Preparation time: 5 minutes | Cooking time: 8 minutes | Servings: 4

Ingredients:

- 1 cup canned artichoke hearts, drained
- 1 pound smoked salmon, skinless, boneless and cubed
- 1 tablespoon olive oil
- A pinch of salt and black pepper
- 1 cup cherry tomatoes, cubed
- ¼ cup coconut cream
- 1 tablespoon chives, chopped

Directions:

In your instant pot, mix the artichoke hearts with the salmon and the rest of the ingredients, toss, put the lid on and cook on High for 8 minutes. Release the pressure fast for 5 minutes, divide the mix into small bowls and serve as an appetizer.

Nutrition: calories 206, fat 12.4, fiber 0.9, carbs 2.6, protein 21.5

Salmon and Cod Cakes

Preparation time: 10 minutes | Cooking time: 10 minutes | Servings: 4

Ingredients:

- 1 tablespoon olive oil
- 1 egg, whisked
- 1 cup tomato passata
- 4 tablespoons almond flour
- ½ pound cod fillets, boneless and chopped
- 1 pound salmon meat, minced
- 1 tablespoon parsley, chopped
- 2 tablespoons lime zest
- A pinch of salt and black pepper

Directions:

In a bowl, combine the cod and salmon meat with the rest of the ingredients except the oil and tomato passata, stir and shape medium cakes out of this mix. Set your instant pot on sauté mode, add the oil, heat it up, add the patties and cook them for 2 minutes on each side. Add the tomato passata, put the lid on and cook on High for 8 minutes. Release the pressure naturally for 10 minutes, arrange the cakes on a platter and serve as an appetizer.

Nutrition: calories 62, fat 4.7, fiber 1.3, carbs 3.9, protein 2.3

Green Beans and Cod Salad

Preparation time: 10 minutes | Cooking time: 15 minutes | Servings: 4

Ingredients:

- 1 pound cod fillets, skinless, boneless and cubed
- 2 tablespoons parsley, chopped
- 2 teaspoons lime juice
- 2 cups green beans, trimmed and halved
- A pinch of salt and black pepper
- 1 cup coconut cream
- 1 tablespoon oregano, chopped
- 1 tablespoon chives, chopped

Directions:

In your instant pot, combine the cod with the green beans and the rest of the ingredients except the oregano and chives, put the lid on and cook on High for 15 minutes. Release the pressure naturally for 10 minutes, divide the mix into small bowls, sprinkle the oregano and the chives on top and serve as an appetizer.

Nutrition: calories 160, fat 14.5, fiber 3.8, carbs 8.1, protein 2.6

Shrimp and Leeks Platter

Preparation time: 5 minutes | Cooking time: 5 minutes | Servings: 6

Ingredients:

- 2 pounds shrimp, peeled and deveined
- 2 leeks, sliced
- 1 tablespoon sweet paprika
- 1 tablespoon olive oil
- 1 tablespoon chives, chopped
- ½ cup veggie stock
- 2 garlic cloves, minced

Directions:

Set instant pot on Sauté mode, add the oil, heat it up, add the leeks and garlic and sauté for 1 minute. Add the rest of the ingredients except the chives, put the lid on and cook on High for 4 minutes. Release the pressure fast for 5 minutes, arrange the shrimp and leeks on a platter and serve as an appetizer.

Nutrition: calories 224, fat 5.1, fiber 1, carbs 3.9, protein 35.1

Balsamic Mussels Bowls

Preparation time: 10 minutes | Cooking time: 10 minutes | Servings: 4

Ingredients:

- 2 cups tomato passata
- 2 pounds mussels, scrubbed
- 2 chili peppers, chopped
- ¼ cup veggie stock
- 1 tablespoon olive oil
- ¼ cup balsamic vinegar
- 2 garlic cloves, minced
- A pinch of salt and black pepper
- ½ cup oregano, chopped

Directions:

Set your instant pot on Sauté mode, add oil heat it up, add the chili peppers and the garlic and cook for 2 minutes. Add the rest of the ingredients, put the lid on and cook on High for 8 minutes. Release the pressure naturally for 10 minutes, divide the mix into bowls and serve as an appetizer.

Nutrition: calories 306, fat 9.8, fiber 4.8, carbs 6.5, protein 20.5

Tomato and Zucchini Salsa

Preparation time: 10 minutes | Cooking time: 10 minutes | Servings: 4

Ingredients:
- 1 pound tomatoes, cubed
- 2 zucchinis, cubed
- 2 tablespoons olive oil
- ¼ cup chicken stock
- ½ teaspoon red pepper flakes
- 2 teaspoons garlic, minced
- 2 teaspoons ginger, chopped
- 1 tablespoon cilantro, chopped
- 2 teaspoons oregano, dried

Directions:

Set your instant pot on Sauté mode, add the oil, heat it up, add the pepper flakes, garlic and ginger and sauté for 2 minutes. Add the rest of the ingredients, put the lid on and cook on High for 8 minutes. Release the pressure naturally for 10 minutes, divide the salsa into bowls and serve cold.

Nutrition: calories 105, fat 7.6, fiber 3, carbs 6.7, protein 2.5

Sweet Shrimp Bowls

Preparation time: 5 minutes | Cooking time: 5 minutes | Servings: 6

Ingredients:
- 2 pounds shrimp, peeled and deveined
- 2 scallions, chopped
- 1 cup veggie stock
- 1 tablespoon olive oil
- 2 garlic cloves, minced
- 1 avocado, peeled, pitted and cubed
- 1 tablespoon sweet paprika

Directions:

Set your instant pot on Sauté mode, add the oil, heat it up, add the scallions and the ginger, stir and cook for 1 minute. Add the rest of the ingredients, put the lid on and cook on High for 4 minutes. Release the pressure fast for 5 minutes, divide the mix into bowls and serve as an appetizer.

Nutrition: calories 274, fat 11.6, fiber 2.8, carbs 6.5, protein 35.4

Parsley Clams Platter

Preparation time: 10 minutes | Cooking time: 12 minutes | Servings: 4

Ingredients:

- 20 clams, scrubbed
- 2 spring onions, chopped
- 1 and ½ cups veggie stock
- 2 tablespoons parsley, chopped
- 2 teaspoons lime zest, grated
- 1 tablespoon lime juice

Directions:

In your instant pot, combine the clams with the stock and the rest of the ingredients, put the lid on and cook on High for 12 minutes. Release the pressure naturally for 10 minutes, arrange the clams on a platter and serve.

Nutrition: calories 224, fat 4.5, fiber 1.2, carbs 2.7, protein 1.3

Zucchinis and Walnuts Salsa

Preparation time: 10 minutes | Cooking time: 12 minutes | Servings: 4

Ingredients:

- 4 zucchinis, sliced
- ½ cup veggie stock
- 3 garlic cloves, minced
- 1 tablespoon ghee, melted
- 1 cup walnuts, chopped
- ¼ cup parsley, chopped
- ¼ cup parmesan cheese, grated
- 1 teaspoon oregano, dried
- 1 teaspoon balsamic vinegar

Directions:

In your instant pot, combine the zucchinis with the stock and the rest of the ingredients except the parmesan, put the lid on and cook on High for 12 minutes. Release the pressure naturally for 10 minutes, divide the mix into bowls, sprinkle the parmesan on top and serve as an appetizer.

Nutrition: calories 259, fat 22.1, fiber 4.6, carbs 5.9, protein 10.2

Shrimp and Beef Bowls
Preparation time: 10 minutes | **Cooking time:** 10 minutes | **Servings:** 4

Ingredients:

- 1 and ½ pounds shrimp, peeled and deveined
- ½ pound beef, cut into strips
- 1 tablespoon Italian seasoning
- 1 cup chicken stock
- A pinch of salt and black pepper
- 1 tablespoon olive oil
- 1 tablespoon sweet paprika
- 1 tablespoon cilantro, chopped
- 1 teaspoon red pepper flakes, crushed

Directions:

Set the instant pot on Sauté mode, add the oil, heat it up, add the beef and brown for 2 minutes. Add the rest of the ingredients, put the lid on and cook on High for 8 minutes. Release the pressure naturally fro 10 minutes, divide the mix into bowls and serve as an appetizer.

Nutrition: calories 155, fat 8.5, fiber 0.8, carbs 1.8, protein 17.7

Coconut Shrimp Platter
Preparation time: 10 minutes | Cooking time: 4 minutes | Servings: 4

Ingredients:

- 2 pounds shrimp, peeled and deveined
- 2 tablespoons coconut aminos
- 3 tablespoons balsamic vinegar
- ¾ cup veggie stock
- 1 tablespoon chives, chopped
- 1 tablespoon basil, chopped
- 1 tablespoon chervil, chopped

Directions:

In your instant pot, combine the shrimp with the aminos and the rest of the ingredients, put the lid on and cook on High for 5 minutes. Release the pressure naturally for 10 minutes, arrange the shrimp on a platter and serve.

Nutrition: calories 273, fat 3.9, fiber 0.1, carbs 3.8, protein 17.8

Marinated Shrimp
Preparation time: 10 minutes | Cooking time: 6 minutes | Servings: 4

Ingredients:
- 1 and ½ pounds shrimp, peeled and deveined
- ¼ cup chicken stock
- 1 tablespoon avocado oil
- Juice of ½ lemon
- 4 garlic cloves, minced
- 2 thyme springs, chopped
- 1 tablespoon rosemary, chopped
- Salt and black pepper to the taste

Directions:
In your instant pot, combine the shrimp with the stock and the rest of the ingredients, put the lid on and cook on High for 6 minutes. Release the pressure naturally for 10 minutes, arrange the shrimp on a platter and serve as an appetizer.

Nutrition: calories 282, fat 4.5, fiber 0.6, carbs 2.3, protein 30.4

Eggplant and Spinach Dip
Preparation time: 10 minutes | Cooking time: 15 minutes | Servings: 4

Ingredients:
- 2 eggplants, cubed
- 1 cup baby spinach
- ¼ cup veggie stock
- ¼ cup coconut cream
- A pinch of salt and black pepper
- 2 garlic cloves, minced
- 1 tablespoon lemon juice

Directions:
In your instant pot, combine the eggplants with the spinach and the rest of the ingredients, put the lid on and cook on High for 15 minutes. Release the pressure naturally for 10 minutes, blend the mix with an immersion blender, divide into bowls and serve as a party dip.

Nutrition: calories 108, fat 4.1, fiber 2.6, carbs 3.7, protein 3.5

Balsamic Endives

Preparation time: 10 minutes | Cooking time: 12 minutes | Servings: 4

Ingredients:

- 4 endives, trimmed and halved lengthwise
- A pinch of salt and black pepper
- 2 tablespoons lime juice
- ¼ cup olive oil
- 2 teaspoons balsamic vinegar
- 1 teaspoon thyme, dried
- 2 cups water

Directions:

Put the water in the instant pot, add steamer basket, add the endives inside, put the lid on and cook on High for 12 minutes. Release the pressure naturally for 10 minutes, transfer the endives to a bowl, add the rest of the ingredients, toss gently, arrange everything on a platter and serve.

Nutrition: calories 109, fat 12.6, fiber 0.1, carbs 0.2, protein 1

Italian Asparagus

Preparation time: 4 minutes | Cooking time: 4 minutes | Servings: 4

Ingredients:

- 1 cup water
- 1 pound asparagus, trimmed
- ½ tablespoon Italian seasoning
- A pinch of salt and black pepper
- 1 tablespoon cilantro, chopped
- 1 tablespoon lemon juice
- 1 teaspoon olive oil

Directions:

Put the water in your instant pot, add steamer basket, add the asparagus, put the lid on and cook on High for 4 minutes. Release the pressure fast for 4 minutes, transfer the asparagus to a bowl, add the rest of the ingredients, toss, arrange everything on a platter and serve.

Nutrition: calories 39, fat 2.1, fiber 1.1, carbs 1.3, protein 2.5

Fennel and Leeks Platter

Preparation time: 5 minutes | Cooking time: 8 minutes | Servings: 4

Ingredients:

- 4 leeks, roughly sliced
- 2 fennel bulbs, halved
- 1 tablespoon smoked paprika
- 1 teaspoon chili sauce
- A pinch of salt and black pepper
- 1 tablespoon ghee, melted
- ½ cup chicken stock

Directions:

In your instant pot, combine the leeks with the fennel, salt, pepper and the stock, put the lid on and cook on High for 8 minutes. Release the pressure fast for 5 minutes, arrange the leeks and fennel on a platter, sprinkle the paprika on top, drizzle the chili sauce and the ghee and serve as an appetizer.

Nutrition: calories 124, fat 4, fiber 2.1, carbs 3.3, protein 3.2

Nutmeg Endives

Preparation time: 10 minutes | Cooking time: 10 minutes | Servings: 4

Ingredients:

- 4 endives, trimmed and halved
- 1 cup water
- Salt and black pepper to the taste
- 2 tablespoons olive oil
- 1 teaspoon nutmeg, ground
- 1 tablespoon chives, chopped

Directions:

Add the water to your instant pot, add steamer basket, add the endives inside, put the lid on and cook on High for 10 minutes. Release the pressure naturally for 10 minutes, arrange the endives on a platter, drizzle the oil, season with salt, pepper and nutmeg, sprinkle the chives at the end and serve as an appetizer.

Nutrition: calories 63, fat 7.2, fiber 0.1, carbs 0.3, protein 0.1

Thyme Eggplants and Celery Spread

Preparation time: 10 minutes | Cooking time: 12 minutes | Servings: 4

Ingredients:

- 2 pounds eggplant, roughly chopped
- A pinch of salt and black pepper
- 2 celery stalks, chopped
- 2 tablespoons olive oil
- 4 garlic cloves, minced
- ½ cup veggie stock
- 2 tablespoons lime juice
- 1 bunch thyme, chopped

Directions:

Set your instant pot on sauté mode, add the oil, heat it up, add the celery stalks and the garlic and sauté for 2 minutes. Add the rest of the ingredients, put the lid on and cook on High for 10 minutes. Release the pressure naturally for 10 minutes, blend the mix using an immersion blender, divide into cups and serve as a spread.

Nutrition: calories 123, fat 7.4, fiber 1.8, carbs 3.7, protein 2.5

Shrimp and Okra Bowls

Preparation time: 10 minutes | Cooking time: 12 minutes | Servings: 4

Ingredients:

- 1 pound okra, trimmed
- ½ pound shrimp, peeled and deveined
- A pinch of salt and black pepper
- 2 tablespoons olive oil
- 1 cup tomato passata, chopped
- 1 tablespoon cilantro, chopped

Directions:

In your instant pot, combine the okra with the shrimp and the rest of the ingredients, put the lid on and cook on High for 12 minutes. Release the pressure fast for 5 minutes, divide the mix into bowls and serve as an appetizer.

Nutrition: calories 188, fat 8.3, fiber 4.6, carbs 6.1, protein 15.6

Mushrooms Salsa

Preparation time: 10 minutes | Cooking time: 10 minutes | Servings: 4

Ingredients:

- 1 pound white mushrooms, halved
- A pinch of salt and black pepper
- 1 tablespoon ghee, melted
- ¼ cup chicken stock
- 1 tablespoon rosemary, chopped
- 1 tablespoon basil, chopped
- 1 tablespoon oregano, chopped
- 2 tomatoes, cubed
- 1 avocado, peeled, pitted and cubed

Directions:

In your instant pot, combine the mushrooms with salt, pepper and the rest of the ingredients, put the lid on and cook on High for 10 minutes. Release the pressure naturally for 10 minutes, divide the salsa into bowls and serve as an appetizer.

Nutrition: calories 173, fat 13.7, fiber 6.2, carbs 7.7, protein 5.3

Cheesy Mushroom and Tomato Salad

Preparation time: 10 minutes | Cooking time: 10 minutes | Servings: 4

Ingredients:

- 4 tomatoes, cubed
- ½ cup veggie stock
- A pinch of salt and black pepper
- 1 tablespoon ghee, melted
- 1 pound mushrooms, halved
- 1 cup mozzarella, shredded
- 1 tablespoon parsley, chopped

Directions:

Set your instant pot on sauté mode, add the ghee, heat it up, add the mushrooms, stir and sauté for 2 minutes. Add the rest of the ingredients except the mozzarella and toss. Sprinkle the mozzarella on top, put the lid on and cook on High for 8 minutes. Release the pressure naturally for 10 minutes, divide the mix into bowls and serve as an appetizer.

Nutrition: calories 95, fat 5, fiber 2.3, carbs 4.7, protein 6.7

Olives Spread

Preparation time: 10 minutes | Cooking time: 15 minutes | Servings: 4

Ingredients:

- 2 cups black olives, pitted and haled
- 2 garlic cloves, minced
- 1 tablespoon lemon juice
- 1 tablespoon olive oil
- A pinch of salt and black pepper
- 1 tablespoon parsley, chopped
- ¼ cup chicken stock

Directions:

In your instant pot, combine the black olives with the stock, salt and the rest of the ingredients, put the lid on and cook on High for 10 minutes. Release the pressure naturally for 10 minutes, blend the mix using an immersion blender, divide into bowls and serve as a party spread.

Nutrition: calories 111, fat 10.8, fiber 2.2, carbs 4.9, protein 0.8

Basil Stuffed Bell Peppers

Preparation time: 10 minutes | Cooking time: 15 minutes | Servings: 4

Ingredients:

- 4 red bell peppers, tops cut off and deseeded
- 2 tablespoons parsley, chopped
- 2 cups basil, chopped
- ¼ cup mozzarella, shredded
- 1 tablespoon garlic, minced
- 2 teaspoons lemon juice
- 1 cup baby spinach, torn
- 2 cups water

Directions:

In a bowl, mix all the ingredients except the water and the peppers, stir well and stuff the peppers with this mix. Add the water to your instant pot, add the trivet inside, arrange the bell peppers in the pot, put the lid on and cook on High for 15 minutes. Release the pressure naturally for 10 minutes, arrange the peppers on a platter and serve as an appetizer.

Nutrition: calories 52, fat 4.8, fiber 2.4, carbs 3.6, protein 2.5

Mussels Salad

Preparation time: 10 minutes | Cooking time: 6 minutes | Servings: 4

Ingredients:

- 1 pound mussels, scrubbed
- 2 cups baby spinach
- ½ cup chicken stock
- 1 tablespoon balsamic vinegar
- 2 scallions, chopped
- ½ teaspoon olive oil
- ½ teaspoon chili powder
- ½ teaspoon oregano, chopped
- A pinch of salt and black pepper

Directions:

In your instant pot, mix the mussels with the stock, salt and pepper, put the lid on and cook on High for 6 minutes. Release the pressure naturally for 10 minutes, transfer the mussels to a bowl, add the rest of the ingredients, toss, and serve as an appetizer.

Nutrition: calories 112, fat 3.4, fiber 0.7, carbs 1.7, protein 14.1

Oregano Beef Bites
Preparation time: 10 minutes | Cooking time: 15 minutes | Servings: 4

Ingredients:
- 1 tablespoon lime juice
- 2 tablespoons avocado oil
- 1 pound beef stew meat, cubed
- 2 garlic cloves, minced
- 1 tablespoon smoked paprika
- 1 tablespoon oregano, chopped
- 1 tablespoon lime zest, grated
- 1 cup beef stock

Directions:
Set the instant pot on Sauté mode, add the oil, heat it up, add the meat and brown for 5 minutes. Add the rest of the ingredients, put the lid on and cook on High for 10 minutes. Release the pressure naturally for 10 minutes, arrange the beef bites on a platter and serve.

Nutrition: calories 236, fat 8.4, fiber 1.6, carbs 2.8, protein 34.5

Watercress and Zucchini Salsa
Preparation time: 5 minutes | Cooking time: 12 minutes | Servings: 4

Ingredients:
- 1 bunch watercress, trimmed
- Juice of 1 lime
- ¼ cup chicken stock
- 2 teaspoons thyme, dried
- 2 tablespoons avocado oil
- 1 cup tomato, cubed
- 1 avocado, peeled, pitted and cubed
- 2 zucchinis, cubed
- 2 spring onions, chopped
- 3 garlic cloves, minced
- ¼ cup cilantro, chopped
- 1 tablespoon balsamic vinegar

Directions:
Set the instant pot on Sauté mode, add the oil, heat it up, add the garlic and sauté for 2 minutes. Add the rest of the ingredients, put the lid on and cook on High for 10 minutes. Release the pressure fast for 5 minutes, divide the salsa into cups and serve as an appetizer.

Nutrition: calories 144, fat 11.1, fiber 4.4, carbs 5.3, protein

Basil Shallots and Peppers Dip

Preparation time: 5 minutes | Cooking time: 15 minutes | Servings: 2

Ingredients:

- ½ cup lemon juice
- 3 shallots, minced
- ½ teaspoon hot sauce
- 1 tablespoon balsamic vinegar
- 1 and ½ pounds mixed peppers, roughly chopped
- ¼ cup chicken stock
- 1 tablespoon olive oil
- 2 tablespoons basil, chopped

Directions:

Set the instant pot on Sauté mode, add the oil, heat it up, add the shallots and sauté for 2 minutes. Add the rest of the ingredients, put the lid on and cook on High for 13 minutes. Release the pressure fast for 5 minutes, blend the mix using an immersion blender, divide into bowls and serve.

Nutrition: calories 78, fat 7.6, fiber 0.3, carbs 1.5, protein 0.7

Olives and Spinach Dip

Preparation time: 5 minutes | Cooking time: 10 minutes | Servings: 4

Ingredients:

- 4 cups baby spinach
- ½ cup coconut cream
- A pinch of salt and black pepper
- 2 tablespoons avocado oil
- 4 garlic cloves, roasted and minced
- 2 tablespoons lime juice
- 1 tablespoon chives, chopped
- 1 cup kalamata olives, pitted and halved

Directions:

In your instant pot, combine all the ingredients except the chives, put the lid on and cook on High for 10 minutes. Release the pressure fast for 5 minutes, blend the mix using an immersion blender, add chives, stir, divide into bowls and serve as a party dip.

Nutrition: calories 129, fat 11.8, fiber 2.8, carbs 6.3, protein 2.1

Mint Salmon and Radish Salad

Preparation time: 10 minutes | Cooking time: 15 minutes | Servings: 4

Ingredients:

- 1 pound salmon fillets, boneless, skinless and cubed
- 2 cups red radishes, sliced
- 1 shallot, sliced
- ½ tablespoons avocado oil
- 2 tablespoons mint leaves, chopped
- ½ cup coconut cream
- A pinch of salt and black pepper

Directions:

Set the instant pot on Sauté mode, add the oil, heat it up, add the shallot and sauté for 2 minutes. Add the salmon and cook for 2 minutes more. Add the rest of the ingredients, put the lid on and cook on High for 10 minutes. Release the pressure naturally for 10 minutes, divide the mix into bowls and serve as an appetizer.

Nutrition: calories 232, fat 14.5, fiber 1.9, carbs 4, protein 23.2

Red Chard Spread

Preparation time: 10 minutes | Cooking time: 15 minutes | Servings: 4

Ingredients:

- 1 pound red chard
- 1 cup spring onions, chopped
- 1 cup veggie stock
- 1 tablespoon sweet paprika
- 1 tablespoon lime juice
- 2 tablespoons olive oil
- 2 garlic cloves, minced
- ½ cup coconut cream
- 1 tablespoon chives, chopped

Directions:

In your instant pot, combine chard with the rest of the ingredients except the cream and the chives, put the lid on and cook on High for 15 minutes. Release the pressure naturally for 10 minutes, add the cream, blend everything using an immersion blender, divide into bowls, sprinkle the chives on top and serve.

Nutrition: calories 144, fat 14.4, fiber 2, carbs 5, protein 1.5

Salmon and Swiss Chard Salad

Preparation time: 10 minutes | Cooking time: 15 minutes | Servings: 4

Ingredients:

- 1 teaspoon olive oil
- 1 pound salmon fillets, boneless, skinless and cubed
- A pinch of salt and black pepper
- ¼ pound Swiss chard, torn
- 1 tablespoon rosemary, chopped
- 1 tablespoon lime juice
- 1 spring onion, chopped
- ¼ cup chicken stock

Directions:

Set the instant pot on Sauté mode, add the oil, heat it up, add the spring onion and sauté for 2 minutes. Add the salmon and cook for 2 minutes on each side. Add the rest of the ingredients, put the lid on and cook on High for 10 minutes. Release the pressure naturally for 10 minutes, divide the mix into bowls and serve as an appetizer.

Nutrition: calories 170, fat 8.4, fiber 0.9, carbs 1.9, protein 22.7

Basil Peppers Salsa

Preparation time: 10 minutes | Cooking time: 12 minutes | Servings: 4

Ingredients:

- 1 and ½ pounds mixed bell peppers, cut into strips
- 2 tablespoons parsley, chopped
- 2 tablespoons basil, chopped
- 2 teaspoons lime juice
- 1 tablespoon avocado oil
- ½ cup tomato passata
- 2 tomatoes, cubed
- 1 avocado, peeled, pitted and cubed
- A pinch of salt and black pepper

Directions:

In your instant pot, combine all the ingredients, put the lid on and cook on High for 12 minutes. Release the pressure naturally for 10 minutes, transfer the mix to small bowls, toss and serve as an appetizer.

Nutrition: calories 127, fat 10.5, fiber 4.8, carbs 7.8, protein 2

Pesto Chicken Salad

Preparation time: 10 minutes | Cooking time: 20 minutes | Servings: 4

Ingredients:

- 1 pound chicken breast, skinless, boneless and cubed
- 2 tablespoons basil pesto
- 2 tablespoons olive oil
- 2 spring onions, chopped
- 2 tablespoons garlic, chopped
- 1 cup chicken stock
- 1 cup tomatoes, crushed
- 1 tablespoon oregano, chopped

Directions:

Set your instant pot on Sauté mode, add the oil, heat it up, add the chicken and the onions and brown for 5 minutes. Add the rest of the ingredients except the basil, put the lid on and cook on High for 15 minutes. Release the pressure naturally for 10 minutes, divide the mix into bowls and serve right away.

Nutrition: calories 212, fat 10.2, fiber 1.3, carbs 4.6, protein 25.2

Cabbage and Spinach Slaw

Preparation time: 10 minutes | Cooking time: 15 minutes | Servings: 4

Ingredients:

- 2 cups red cabbage, shredded
- 1 tablespoon avocado mayonnaise
- 1 spring onion, chopped
- 1 pound baby spinach
- ½ cup chicken stock
- 1 teaspoon chili powder
- 1 tablespoon sweet paprika
- 1 tablespoon chives, chopped
- 1 tablespoon avocado oil

Directions:

Set instant pot on Sauté mode, add the oil, heat it up, add the onion and cook for 2 minutes. Add the rest of the ingredients except the spinach, avocado mayonnaise and the chives, put the lid on and cook on High for 12 minutes. Release the pressure naturally for 10 minutes, transfer the mix to a bowl, add the remaining ingredients, toss and serve as an appetizer.

Nutrition: calories 72, fat 3.8, fiber 1.2, carbs 2.6, protein 4.3

Cabbage, Tomato and Avocado Salsa
Preparation time: 5 minutes | Cooking time: 12 minutes | Servings: 4

Ingredients:
- 1 and ½ pound cherry tomatoes, cubed
- ¼ cup veggie stock
- 2 tablespoons olive oil
- ¼ cup balsamic vinegar
- 2 spring onions, chopped
- 1 red cabbage head, shredded
- 1 tablespoon basil, chopped
- 1 tablespoon parsley, chopped
- 1 tablespoon chives, chopped
- 1 avocado, peeled, pitted and cubed

Directions:

In your instant pot, combine the tomatoes the rest of the ingredients, put the lid on and cook on High for 12 minutes. Release the pressure fast for 5 minutes, transfer the mix to small bowls and serve as an appetizer.

Nutrition: calories 254, fat 17.3, fiber 2.5, carbs 5.5, protein 5.4

Shrimp and Mussels Salad
Preparation time: 6 minutes | Cooking time: 12 minutes | Servings: 4

Ingredients:
- 1 pound mussels, scrubbed
- ½ cup tomato passata
- ¼ cup chicken stock
- 1 pound shrimp, peeled and deveined
- 1 and ½ cups baby spinach
- 2 tablespoons olive oil
- 1 teaspoon hot paprika
- 2 teaspoons oregano, dried
- 1 tablespoon parsley, chopped

Directions:

In your instant pot, combine the mussels with the rest of the ingredients except the parsley and the spinach, put the lid on and cook on High for 10 minutes. Release the pressure fast for 6 minutes, set the pot on Sauté mode again, add the spinach and the parsley, toss, cook for 2 minutes more, divide into bowls and serve as an appetizer.

Nutrition: calories 303, fat 11.7, fiber 0.8, carbs 7.8, protein 39.3

Beef, Arugula and Olives Salad

Preparation time: 10 minutes | Cooking time: 20 minutes | Servings: 4

Ingredients:

- 1 and ½ pounds beef, cut into strips
- 2 tomatoes, cubed
- ¼ cup beef stock
- ½ cup black olives, pitted and sliced
- 1 tablespoon avocado oil
- 2 spring onions, chopped
- ½ cup cilantro chopped
- 2 cups tomatoes, chopped
- 1 tablespoon basil, chopped
- A pinch of salt and black pepper
- 1 cup baby arugula

Directions:

Set your instant pot on Sauté mode, add the oil, heat it up, add the onions and the meat and brown for 5 minutes. Add the rest of the ingredients except the arugula, put the lid on and cook on High for 15 minutes. Release the pressure naturally for 10 minutes, transfer the mix to a bowl, add the arugula, toss and serve as an appetizer.

Nutrition: calories 378, fat 16.7, fiber 2.8, carbs 7.8, protein 24.3

Bacon Radish and Shrimp Salad

Preparation time: 5 minutes | Cooking time: 15 minutes | Servings: 4

Ingredients:

- 1 pound shrimp, peeled and deveined
- 1 shallot, chopped
- 2 cups radishes, sliced
- 1 cup bacon, cooked and crumbled
- 1 tablespoon olive oil
- 1 teaspoon sweet paprika
- 1 tablespoon oregano, chopped
- A pinch of salt and black pepper
- 1 cup veggie stock

Directions:

Set your instant pot on Sauté mode, add the oil, heat it up, add the shallot and sauté for 2 minutes. Add the rest of the ingredients except the oregano and the bacon, put the lid on and cook on High for 13 minutes. Release the pressure fast for 5 minutes, transfer the mix to small bowls, sprinkle the oregano and the bacon on top and serve as an appetizer.

Nutrition: calories 179, fat 5.7, fiber 1.6, carbs 4.5, protein 26.5

Cheesy Radish Spread

Preparation time: 10 minutes | Cooking time: 10 minutes | Servings: 4

Ingredients:

- 2 cups radishes, sliced
- 4 ounces cream cheese, soft
- 1 cup cheddar cheese, grated
- ½ cup chicken stock
- ½ cup coconut cream
- A pinch of salt and black pepper
- 2 shallots, minced
- 1 teaspoon sweet paprika

Directions:

In your instant pot, combine all the ingredients, stir, put the lid on and cook on High for 12 minutes. Release the pressure naturally for 10 minutes, blend everything using an immersion blender, divide into bowls and serve.

Nutrition: calories 294, fat 20.6, fiber 1.8, carbs 5.4, protein 10.4

Ketogenic Instant Pot Fish and Seafood Recipes

Cod and Tomatoes
Preparation time: 10 minutes | Cooking time: 15 minutes | Servings: 4

Ingredients:

- 4 cod fillets, boneless and skinless
- ¼ cup chicken stock
- 2 tablespoons olive oil
- Juice of 1 lemon
- 2 shallots, chopped
- 3 tomatoes, cubed
- 4 thyme springs, chopped
- A pinch of salt and black pepper

Directions:

Set the instant pot on Sauté mode, add the oil, heat it up, add the shallots and cook for 2 minutes. Add the rest of the ingredients, put the lid on and cook on High for 12 minutes. Release the pressure naturally for 10 minutes, divide everything between plates and serve.

Nutrition: calories 232, fat 16.5, fiber 1.1, carbs 4.8, protein 16.5

Cod and Cilantro Sauce
Preparation time: 5 minutes | Cooking time: 15 minutes | Servings: 4

Ingredients:

- 4 cod fillets, boneless
- ¼ cup chicken stock
- 1 tablespoon ghee, melted
- 1 tablespoon ginger, grated
- Salt and black pepper to the taste
- Juice of 1lemon
- 2 tablespoons cilantro, chopped

Directions:

In a blender, combine the ghee with the ginger, lemon juice and cilantro and blend well. In your instant pot, combine the cod with the cilantro sauce, salt, pepper and the stock, put the lid on and cook on High for 15 minutes. Release the pressure fast for 5 minutes, divide everything between plates and serve.

Nutrition: calories 188, fat 12.8, fiber 0.2, carbs 2.2, protein 16.8

Salmon and Black Olives Mix

Preparation time: 5 minutes | Cooking time: 15 minutes | Servings: 4

Ingredients:

- 1 pound salmon fillets, boneless, skinless and cubed
- 1 cup black olives, pitted and chopped
- 1 cup kalamata olives, pitted and chopped
- 2 garlic cloves, minced
- 1 tablespoon olive oil
- A pinch of salt and black pepper
- ¼ cup chicken stock
- 1 tablespoon parsley, chopped

Directions:

Set the instant pot on Sauté mode, add the oil, heat it up, add the fish and sear for 2 minutes on each side. Add the rest of the ingredients, put the lid on and cook on High for 10 minutes. Release the pressure fast for 5 minutes, divide everything between plates and serve.

Nutrition: calories 261, fat 17.6, fiber 2.2, carbs 4.8, protein 22.5

Coriander Cod Mix

Preparation time: 5 minutes | Cooking time: 15 minutes | Servings: 4

Ingredients:

- 4 cod fillets, boneless and skinless
- 1 cup coconut cream
- 2 spring onions, sliced
- 2 garlic cloves, minced
- 1 tablespoons coriander, chopped
- A pinch of salt and black pepper
- 2 tablespoons lime juice

Directions:

In your instant pot, combine the trout with the cream and the rest of the ingredients, put the lid on and cook on High for 15 minutes. Release the pressure fast for 5 minutes, divide everything between plates and serve.

Nutrition: calories 297, fat 24.3, fiber 1.6, carbs 5.4, protein 17.6

Cod and Zucchinis

Preparation time: 5 minutes | Cooking time: 15 minutes | Servings: 4

Ingredients:

- 4 cod fillets, boneless and skinless
- 2 zucchinis, sliced
- 1 tablespoon avocado oil
- 2 garlic cloves, minced
- 1 tablespoon sweet paprika
- Salt and black pepper to the taste
- 1 tablespoon parsley, chopped
- ½ cup veggie stock

Directions:

Set the instant pot on Sauté mode, add the oil, heat it up, add the garlic and sauté for 2 minutes. Add the rest of the ingredients, put the lid on and cook on High for 12 minutes. Release the pressure naturally for 5 minutes, divide the mix between plates and serve.

Nutrition: calories 182, fat 10.4, fiber 1.9, carbs 6.2, protein 17.5

Paprika Trout

Preparation time: 5 minutes | Cooking time: 12 minutes | Servings: 4

Ingredients:

- 4 trout fillets, boneless and skinless
- ½ cup chicken stock
- A pinch of salt and black pepper
- ½ teaspoon oregano, dried
- 2 teaspoons sweet paprika
- 1 tablespoon chives, chopped

Directions:

In your instant pot, combine the trout with the rest of the ingredients, put the lid on and cook on High for 12 minutes. Release the pressure fast for 5 minutes, divide the mix between plates and serve.

Nutrition: calories 132, fat 5.5, fiber 0.5, carbs 0.9, protein 16.8

Lime Shrimp

Preparation time: 5minutes | *Cooking time:* 8 minutes | *Servings:* 4

Ingredients:

- 1 pound shrimp, peeled and deveined
- Zest of 1 lime, grated
- Juice of 1 lime
- 1 cup chicken stock
- ¼ cup cilantro, chopped
- A pinch of salt and black pepper

Directions:

In your instant pot, combine the shrimp with the rest of the ingredients, put the lid on and cook on High for 8 minutes. Release the pressure fast for 5 minutes, divide the shrimp between plates and serve with a side salad.

Nutrition: calories 138, fat 3.8, fiber 0, carbs 2, protein 26

Trout and Radishes

Preparation time: 5 minutes | *Cooking time:* 12 minutes | *Servings:* 4

Ingredients:

- 4 trout fillets, boneless and skinless
- A pinch of salt and black pepper
- 1 tablespoon parsley, chopped
- 2 tablespoons tomato passata
- 2 cups red radishes, sliced

Directions:

In your instant pot, combine all the ingredients, put the lid on and cook on High for 12 minutes. Release the pressure fast for 5 minutes, divide everything between plates and serve.

Nutrition: calories 129, fat 5.3, fiber 1.1, carbs 2.5, protein 17

Cod and Broccoli

Preparation time: 5 minutes | *Cooking time:* 15 minutes | *Servings:* 4

Ingredients:

- 4 cod fillets, boneless and skinless
- A pinch of salt and black pepper
- 1 pound broccoli florets
- 2 tablespoon tomato passata
- 1 cup chicken stock
- 1 tablespoon cilantro, chopped

Directions:

In your instant pot, combine all the ingredients, put the lid on and cook on High for 15 minutes. Release the pressure fast for 5 minutes, divide the mix between plates and serve.

Nutrition: calories 197, fat 10, fiber 3.1, carbs 4.3, protein 19.4

Rosemary Trout and Cauliflower

Preparation time: 10 minutes | Cooking time: 15 minutes | Servings: 4

Ingredients:

- 4 trout fillets, boneless and skinless
- ½ cup veggie stock
- 2 garlic cloves, minced
- 2 cups cauliflower florets
- 1 tablespoon avocado oil
- A pinch of salt and black pepper
- 1 tablespoon rosemary, chopped

Directions:

Set the instant pot on Sauté mode, add the oil, heat it up, add the garlic and sauté for 2 minutes. Add the rest of the ingredients, put the lid on and cook on High for 13 minutes. Release the pressure naturally for 10 minutes, divide the mix between plates and serve.

Nutrition: calories 140, fat 5.9, fiber 1.8, carbs 3.9, protein 17.7

Cinnamon Cod Mix

Preparation time: 5 minutes | Cooking time: 12 minutes | Servings: 4

Ingredients:

- 4 cod fillets, boneless and skinless
- 1 tablespoon cinnamon powder
- 1 cup cherry tomatoes, cubed
- Juice of ½ lemon
- ½ cup veggie stock
- A pinch of salt and black pepper
- 1 tablespoon cilantro, chopped

Directions:

In your instant pot, mix the fish with the rest of the ingredients, put the lid on and cook on High for 12 minutes. Release the pressure fast for 5 minutes, divide everything between plates and serve.

Nutrition: calories 162, fat 9.6, fiber 0.3, carbs 3, protein 16.5

Trout and Eggplant Mix

Preparation time: 10 minutes | Cooking time: 15 minutes | Servings: 4

Ingredients:

- 4 trout fillets, boneless
- 2 scallions, chopped
- 2 eggplants, cubed
- ½ cup chicken stock
- 2 tablespoons parsley, chopped
- 3 tablespoons olive oil
- A pinch of salt and black pepper
- 2 tablespoons smoked paprika

Directions:

Set the instant pot on Sauté mode, add the oil, heat it up, add the scallions and the eggplant and cook for 2 minutes, Add the rest of the ingredients except the parsley, put the lid on and cook on High for 13 minutes. Release the pressure naturally for 10 minutes, divide the mix between plates and serve with the parsley sprinkled on top.

Nutrition: calories 291, fat 16.8, fiber 4.5, carbs 6.4, protein 20

Salmon and Tomato Passata

Preparation time: 10 minutes | Cooking time: 15 minutes | Servings: 4

Ingredients:

- 1 tablespoon olive oil
- 4 salmon fillets, boneless, skinless and cubed
- 1 tablespoon rosemary, chopped
- 1 shallot, chopped
- 1 cup tomato passata
- 1 teaspoon chili powder
- 1 tablespoon chives, chopped
- A pinch of salt and black pepper

Directions:

Set the instant pot on Sauté mode, add the oil, heat it up, add the shallot and sauté for 2 minutes. Add the rest of the ingredients, put the lid on and cook on High for 12 minutes. Release the pressure naturally for 10 minutes, divide the mix between plates and serve.

Nutrition: calories 291, fat 16.8, fiber 4.5, carbs 7.4, protein 20

Salmon and Artichokes

Preparation time: 10 minutes | Cooking time: 15 minutes | Servings: 4

Ingredients:

- 1 pound salmon, skinless, boneless and cubed
- 2 spring onions, chopped
- 12 ounces canned artichokes, roughly chopped
- 1 and ½ cups chicken stock
- A pinch of salt and black pepper
- 1 tablespoon cilantro, chopped

Directions:

In your instant pot, combine all the ingredients, put the lid on and cook on High for 15 minutes. Release the pressure naturally for 10 minutes, divide everything between plates and serve.

Nutrition: calories 193, fat 7.1, fiber 4.1, carbs 6.4, protein 24.5

Trout and Spinach Mix

Preparation time: 5 minutes | Cooking time: 15 minutes | Servings: 4

Ingredients:

- 6 trout fillets, boneless
- 2 tablespoons avocado oil
- 2 scallions, minced
- 2 garlic cloves, minced
- 2 tablespoons cilantro, chopped
- 1 cup baby spinach
- A pinch of salt and black pepper
- 2 tablespoons balsamic vinegar

Directions:

Set the instant pot on Sauté mode, add the oil, heat it up, add the scallions and the garlic and sauté for 2 minutes. Add the rest of the ingredients, put the lid on and cook on High for 12 minutes. Release the pressure fast for 5 minutes, divide the mix between plates and serve.

Nutrition: calories 194, fat 8.8, fiber 0.7, carbs 1.8, protein 25.4

Sea Bass and Sauce

Preparation time: 10 minutes | Cooking time: 15 minutes | Servings: 4

Ingredients:

- 4 sea bass fillets, boneless and skinless
- 2 tablespoons lime juice
- 2 garlic cloves, minced
- 1 shallot, chopped
- 1 cup chicken stock
- 1 cup tomato passata
- A pinch of salt and black pepper

Directions:

In your instant pot, combine the fish with the rest of the ingredients, put the lid on and cook on High for 15 minutes. Release the pressure naturally for 10 minutes, divide the mix between plates and serve.

Nutrition: calories 154, fat 2.9, fiber 1.3, carbs 2.5, protein 25

Sea Bass and Pesto
Preparation time: 5 minutes | Cooking time: 12 minutes | Servings: 4

Ingredients:

- 4 sea bass fillets, skinless, boneless
- 2 tablespoons olive oil
- 2 tablespoons garlic, chopped
- 1 cup basil, chopped
- 2 tablespoons pine nuts
- A pinch of salt and black pepper
- 1 cup tomato passata
- 1 tablespoon parsley, chopped

Directions:

In your blender, combine the oil with the garlic, basil, pine nuts, slat and pepper and pulse well. In your instant pot, combine the sea bass with the pesto, salt, pepper, tomato passata and the parsley, put the lid on and cook on High for 12 minutes. Release the pressure fast for 5 minutes, divide the mix between plates and serve.

Nutrition: calories 237, fat 12.7, fiber 1.3, carbs 5.5, protein 25.8

Tuna and Mustard Greens
Preparation time: 10 minutes | Cooking time: 10 minutes | Servings: 4

Ingredients:

- 2 cups mustard greens
- 1 tablespoon olive oil
- 1 cup tomato passata
- 1 shallot, chopped
- 1 tablespoon basil, chopped
- A pinch of salt and black pepper
- 14 ounces tuna fillets, boneless, skinless and cubed

Directions:

Set your instant pot on Sauté mode, add the oil, heat it up, add the shallot and sauté for 2 minutes. Add rest of the ingredients, put the lid on and cook on High for 8 minutes. Release the pressure naturally for 10 minutes, divide the mix between plates and serve.

Nutrition: calories 124, fat 3.7, fiber 1.9, carbs 2.6, protein 1.6

Salmon and Salsa

Preparation time: 10 minutes | Cooking time: 8 minutes | Servings: 4

Ingredients:

- 4 salmon fillets, boneless
- ½ cup veggie stock
- 1 cup black olives, pitted
- 1 cup tomatoes, cubed
- 1 tablespoon basil, chopped
- 1 tablespoon olive oil
- 1 tablespoon balsamic vinegar
- A pinch of salt and black pepper
- 1 tablespoon chives, chopped

Directions:

In your instant pot, combine the fish with the stock, salt and pepper, put the lid on and cook on High for 8 minutes. Release the pressure naturally for 10 minutes and divide the salmon between plates. In a bowl, mix the olives with the rest of the ingredients, toss, add next to the salmon and serve.

Nutrition: calories 313, fat 18.2, fiber 1.7, carbs 4, protein 35.4

Saffron Chili Cod

Preparation time: 5 minutes | Cooking time: 12 minutes | Servings: 4

Ingredients:

- 4 cod fillets, boneless and skinless
- 3 garlic cloves, minced
- 1 teaspoon turmeric powder
- 1 tablespoon chili paste
- 1 cup tomato passata

Directions:

In your instant pot, combine the cod with the rest of the ingredients, put the lid on and cook on High for 12 minutes. Release the pressure fast for 5 minutes, divide everything between plates and serve.

Nutrition: calories 244, fat 12, fiber 1.6, carbs 4.5, protein 14.6

Salmon and Endives

Preparation time: 10 minutes | Cooking time: 15 minutes | Servings: 4

Ingredients:

- 4 salmon fillets, boneless
- 1 cup tomato passata
- 1 shallot, sliced
- 2 endives, trimmed and halved
- 1 tablespoon balsamic vinegar
- A pinch of salt and black pepper
- 1 tablespoon parsley, chopped

Directions:

In your instant pot, combine the salmon with the rest of the ingredients, put the lid on and cook on High for 15 minutes. Release the pressure naturally for 10 minutes, divide the mix between plates and serve.

Nutrition: calories 251, fat 11.1, fiber 1, carbs 3.4, protein 35.4

Chili Tuna

Preparation time: 5 minutes | Cooking time: 15 minutes | Servings: 4

Ingredients:

- 1 pound tuna, skinless, boneless and cubed
- Juice of 1 lemon
- 1 tablespoon chili powder
- 1 cup tomato passata
- A pinch of salt and black pepper
- 1 shallot, chopped
- 1 tablespoon chives, chopped
- 1 tablespoon cilantro, chopped

Directions:

In your instant pot, combine the tuna with the lemon juice and the rest of the ingredients, put the lid on and cook on High for 15 minutes. Release the pressure fast for 5 minutes, divide the chili into bowls and serve.

Nutrition: calories 232, fat 9.6, fiber 1.6, carbs 4.4, protein 31.2

Mackerel and Shrimp Mix

Preparation time: 5 minutes | Cooking time: 12 minutes | Servings: 6

Ingredients:

- 1 pound shrimp, peeled and deveined
- 1 pound mackerel, skinless, boneless and cubed
- 1 cup radishes, cubed
- ½ cup chicken stock
- 2 garlic cloves, minced
- 1 tablespoon olive oil
- 1 cup tomato passata

Directions:

Set instant pot on Sauté mode, add the oil, heat it up, add the radishes and the garlic and sauté for 2 minutes. Add the rest of the ingredients, put the lid on and cook on High for 10 minutes. Release the pressure fast for 5 minutes, divide the mix into bowls and serve.

Nutrition: calories 332, fat 17.4, fiber 0.9, carbs 4.4, protein 36.4

Mackerel and Basil Sauce

Preparation time: 10 minutes | Cooking time: 15 minutes | Servings: 4

Ingredients:

- 1 cup veggie stock
- 2 chili peppers, chopped
- 2 tablespoons olive oil
- 1 pound mackerel, skinless, boneless and cubed
- 2 teaspoons red pepper flakes
- A pinch of salt and black pepper
- ½ cup basil, chopped

Directions:

Set your instant pot on Sauté mode, add the oil, heat it up, add the chili peppers and the pepper flakes and cook for 2 minutes. Add the rest of the ingredients, put the lid on and cook on High for 12 minutes. Release the pressure naturally for 10 minutes, divide everything between plates and serve.

Nutrition: calories 362, fat 14.7, fiber 0.4, carbs 0.8, protein 27.5

Oregano Tuna

Preparation time: 10 minutes | Cooking time: 12 minutes | Servings: 4

Ingredients:

- 1 pound tuna, skinless, boneless and cubed
- 1 cup black olives, pitted and sliced
- 2 tablespoon avocado oil
- 1 shallot, chopped
- 14 ounces tomatoes, chopped
- 2 tablespoons oregano, chopped

Directions:

Set your instant pot on Sauté mode, add the oil, heat it up, add the shallot and sauté for 2 minutes. Add the tuna and the rest of the ingredients, put the lid on and cook on High for 10 minutes. Release the pressure naturally for 10 minutes, divide the mix between plates and serve.

Nutrition: calories 284, fat 14.1, fiber 3.5, carbs 6.7, protein 31.4

Creamy Shrimp and Radish Mix

Preparation time: 5 minutes | Cooking time: 6 minutes | Servings: 4

Ingredients:

- 1 and ½ pound shrimp, peeled and deveined
- 1 cup red radishes, sliced
- ½ cup black olives, pitted
- 2 spring onions, chopped
- 1 and ½ cups coconut cream
- 1 tablespoon cilantro, chopped
- 1 tablespoon sweet paprika

Directions:

In your instant pot, combine the shrimp with the rest of the ingredients, put the lid on and cook on High for 6 minutes. Release the pressure fast for 5 minutes, divide the mix into bowls and serve.

Nutrition: calories 301, fat 5.9, fiber 1.9, carbs 6.4, protein 52.4

Marjoram Tuna

Preparation time: 10 minutes | Cooking time: 15 minutes | Servings: 4

Ingredients:

- 1 and ½ pounds tuna, skinless, boneless and cubed
- 2 spring onions, chopped
- 1 tablespoon avocado oil
- 3 garlic cloves, minced
- ½ cup basil, chopped
- ½ cup chicken stock
- 2 tablespoons tomato passata
- 1 tablespoon marjoram, chopped
- A pinch of salt and black pepper

Directions:

Set your instant pot on Sauté mode, add the oil, heat it up, add the garlic and the spring onions, stir and sauté for 3 minutes. Add the rest of the ingredients, put the lid on and cook on High for 12 minutes. Release the pressure naturally for 10 minutes, divide the mix between plates and serve.

Nutrition: calories 345, fat 16.9, fiber 0.7, carbs 2.4, protein 26.6

Bacon Trout Mix

Preparation time: 10 minutes | Cooking time: 15 minutes | Servings: 4

Ingredients:

- 1 cup bacon, cooked and crumbled
- 4 trout fillets, boneless and skinless
- 10 ounces tomato passata
- 2 tablespoons cilantro, chopped
- 1 shallot, chopped
- 1 tablespoon olive oil
- 1 tablespoon lemon juice

Directions:

Set your instant pot on Sauté mode, add the oil, heat it up, add the shallot and sauté for 2 minutes. Add the rest of the ingredients, put the lid on and cook on High for 13 minutes. Release the pressure naturally for 10 minutes, divide the mix between plates and serve.

Nutrition: calories 166, fat 8.9, fiber 1.1, carbs 3.8, protein 17.5

Tuna and Fennel Mix

Preparation time: 10 minutes | Cooking time: 15 minutes | Servings: 4

Ingredients:

- 1 tablespoon avocado oil
- 1 pound tuna, skinless, boneless and cubed
- 2 tuna fillets, boneless, skinless and cubed
- 3 garlic cloves, minced
- ¼ cup parsley, chopped
- ½ cup chicken stock
- 2 fennel bulbs, sliced
- 1 tablespoon sweet paprika

Directions:

Set the instant pot on Sauté mode, add the oil, heat it up, add the garlic and cook for 2 minutes. Add the tuna, fennel and the rest of the ingredients, put the lid on and cook on High for 13 minutes, Release the pressure naturally for 10 minutes, divide everything between plates and serve.

Nutrition: calories 263, fat 10.2, fiber 2.4, carbs 4.8, protein 23.5

Tilapia Salad

Preparation time: 5 minutes | Cooking time: 12 minutes | Servings: 4

Ingredients:

- 1 and ½ pounds tilapia fillets, boneless, skinless and cubed
- 1 cup black olives, pitted
- 1 cup zucchinis, cubed
- 1 cup baby spinach
- 1 tablespoon olive oil
- 1 tablespoon balsamic vinegar
- A pinch of salt and black pepper
- 2 tomatoes, cubed
- ½ cup chicken stock
- 1 tablespoon lemon juice
- 1 tablespoon sweet paprika

Directions:

In your instant pot, combine the fish with the olives, zucchinis, tomatoes, stock, paprika, salt and pepper, toss, put the lid on and cook on High for 12 minutes. Release the pressure fast for 5 minutes, transfer the mix to a bowl, add the remaining ingredients, toss and serve.

Nutrition: calories 187, fat 8.6, fiber 3, carbs 6.9, protein 22.8

Salmon and Dill Sauce
Preparation time: 10 minutes | Cooking time: 20 minutes | Servings: 6

Ingredients:

- 6 salmon fillets, boneless
- ½ teaspoon lemon pepper
- 1 spring onion, chopped
- Juice of ½ lemon
- A pinch of salt and black pepper
- 1 tablespoon chives, chopped
- ½ cup avocado mayonnaise
- ½ cup heavy cream
- 1 teaspoon dill, chopped

Directions:

Set the instant pot on Sauté mode, add the cream, dill and the rest of the ingredients except the salmon and the mayonnaise, whisk and cook for 5 minutes. Add the fish, put the lid on and cook on High for 15 minutes. Release the pressure naturally for 10 minutes, add the avocado mayonnaise, toss gently, divide everything between plates and serve.

Nutrition: calories 399, fat 22.1, fiber 0.2, carbs 1.1, protein 23.8

Tilapia and Olives Salsa
Preparation time: 10 minutes | Cooking time: 15 minutes | Servings: 4

Ingredients:

- 4 tilapia fillets, boneless
- 1 tablespoon olive oil
- A pinch of salt and black pepper
- 12 ounces tomato passata
- 2 tablespoon sweet red pepper, chopped
- 2 tablespoon green onions, chopped
- ½ tablespoons Italian seasoning
- 1 and ½ cups black olives, pitted
- 1 tablespoon balsamic vinegar

Directions:

Set the instant pot on Sauté mode, add the oil, heat it up, add the fish and cook for 2 minutes on each side. Add salt, pepper and the tomato passata, put the lid on and cook on High for 10 minutes. Release the pressure naturally for 10 minutes and divide the fish between plates. In a bowl, mix the red pepper with the remaining ingredients, toss, divide next to the fish and serve.

Nutrition: calories 155, fat 4.6, fiber 2.5, carbs 3.4, protein 7.4

Catfish and Avocado Mix

Preparation time: 10 minutes | Cooking time: 16 minutes | Servings: 4

Ingredients:

- 4 catfish fillets, boneless
- 2 teaspoons olive oil
- 2 tablespoons lime juice
- 2 tablespoons cilantro, chopped
- A pinch of salt and black pepper
- 2 teaspoons sweet paprika
- 1/3 cup spring onions, chopped
- 2 teaspoons oregano, dried
- 2 teaspoons cumin, dried
- ½ cup tomato passata
- 1 avocado, peeled, pitted and cubed

Directions:

Set the instant pot on Sauté mode, add the oil, heat it up, add the onions and cook for 2 minutes. Add the fish and cook for 1 minute on each side. Add the rest of the ingredients, put the lid on and cook on High for 12 minutes more. Release the pressure naturally for 10 minutes, divide everything between plates and serve.

Nutrition: calories 353, fat 23.4, fiber 2.6, carbs 6.4, protein 15.3

Tilapia and Capers Mix

Preparation time: 10 minutes | Cooking time: 15 minutes | Servings: 4

Ingredients:

- 4 tilapia fillets, boneless
- 3 tablespoons lemon juice
- 2 tablespoons ghee, melted
- A pinch of salt and black pepper
- ½ teaspoon oregano, dried
- 2 tablespoons capers, drained and chopped
- 1 teaspoon sweet paprika
- ½ teaspoon garlic powder
- ½ cup chicken stock

Directions:

Set the instant pot on Sauté mode, add the ghee, melt it, add the fish and sear for 2 minutes on each side. Add salt, pepper and the rest of the ingredients, put the lid on and cook on High for 10 minutes. Release the pressure naturally for 10 minutes, divide the mix between plates and serve.

Nutrition: calories 173, fat 7.2, fiber 0.5, carbs 2.3, protein 4.7

Glazed Salmon

Preparation time: 10 minutes | Cooking time: 15 minutes | Servings: 4

Ingredients:

- 4 salmon fillets, boneless
- A pinch of salt and black pepper
- 4 teaspoons mustard
- 1 tablespoon coconut aminos
- 1 teaspoon balsamic vinegar
- 3 tablespoons swerve

Directions:

Set the instant pot on Sauté mode, add the mustard, the aminos and the rest of the ingredients except the salmon, whisk well and cook for 3 minutes. Add the salmon, put the lid on and cook on High for 12 minutes. Release the pressure naturally for 10 minutes, divide the salmon between plates, drizzle the glaze all over and serve.

Nutrition: calories 251, fat 11.9, fiber 0.5, carbs 1.2, protein 35.4

Spicy Tilapia and Kale

Preparation time: 10 minutes | Cooking time: 20 minutes | Servings: 4

Ingredients:

- 4 tilapia fillets, boneless
- A pinch of salt and black pepper
- 3 tablespoons olive oil
- 2 garlic cloves, minced
- 1 teaspoon fennel seed
- 14 ounces canned tomatoes, crushed
- 1 bunch kale, chopped
- ½ teaspoon red pepper flakes

Directions:

Set the instant pot on Sauté mode, add the oil, heat it up, add the garlic and fennel seed and cook for 3 minutes. Add the rest of the ingredients except the fish, toss and sauté for 4 minutes more. Add the fish, put the lid on and cook on High for 12 minutes. Release the pressure naturally for 10 minutes, divide the mix between plates and serve.

Nutrition: calories 138, fat 11.2, fiber 1.5, carbs 4.8, protein 6.3

Lime Glazed Salmon

Preparation time: 10 minutes | Cooking time: 15 minutes | Servings: 4

Ingredients:

- 4 salmon fillets, boneless
- A pinch of salt and black pepper
- 1 tablespoon ginger, grated
- 1 tablespoon coconut aminos
- 1 tablespoon sesame seeds
- 1 teaspoon lime zest, grated
- 1 tablespoon lime juice
- ½ cup chicken stock

Directions:

Set the instant pot on Sauté mode, add the stock, lime juice and the rest of the ingredients except the salmon and the sesame seeds, whisk and cook for 3 minutes. Add the salmon, put the lid on and cook on High for 12 minutes. Release the pressure naturally for 10 minutes, divide the salmon mix between plates, sprinkle the sesame seeds on top and serve.

Nutrition: calories 255, fat 12.3, fiber 0.5, cabs 1.7, protein 35.4

Tilapia and Zucchini Noodles

Preparation time: 10 minutes | Cooking time: 15 minutes | Servings: 4

Ingredients:

- 4 tilapia fillets, boneless
- ¼ teaspoon garlic powder
- 2 zucchinis, cut with a spiralizer
- ½ teaspoon cumin, ground
- 2 garlic cloves, minced
- ½ teaspoon smoked paprika
- A pinch of salt and black pepper
- 2 teaspoons olive oil
- ½ cup tomato passata

Directions:

Set the instant pot on Sauté mode, add the oil, heat it up, add the garlic, cumin, garlic powder, paprika, salt and pepper, stir and cook for 3 minutes. Add the rest of the ingredients, put the lid on and cook on High for 12 minutes. Release the pressure naturally for 10 minutes, divide the whole mix between plates and serve.

Nutrition: calories 259, fat 13.9, fiber 2.2, carbs 4.9, protein 15.2

Salmon and Coconut Mix

Preparation time: 10 minutes | Cooking time: 20 minutes | Servings: 4

Ingredients:

- 4 salmon fillets, boneless
- 3 tablespoons avocado mayonnaise
- 1 teaspoon lime zest, grated
- ¼ cup coconut cream
- ¼ cup lime juice
- ½ cup coconut, unsweetened and shredded
- 2 teaspoons Cajun seasoning
- A pinch of salt and black pepper

Directions:

Set the instant pot on Sauté mode, add the coconut cream and the rest of the ingredients except the fish, whisk and cook for 5 minutes. Add the fish, put the lid on and cook on High for 10 minutes. Release the pressure naturally for 10 minutes, divide the salmon and the sauce between plates and serve.

Nutrition: calories 306, fat 17.5, fiber 1.4, carbs 2.5, protein 25.3

Haddock and Cilantro Sauce

Preparation time: 10 minutes | Cooking time: 15 minutes | Servings: 4

Ingredients:

- 4 haddock fillets, skinless, boneless and cubed
- 3 teaspoons Italian seasoning
- 2 tablespoons cilantro, chopped
- 2 tomatoes, cubed
- 1 cup heavy cream
- 1 tablespoon lemon juice
- 1 tablespoon avocado oil

Directions:

Set the instant pot on Sauté mode, add the oil, heat it up, add the cilantro, tomatoes, and the rest of the ingredients except the fish, whisk and simmer for 4 minutes. Add the fish, put the lid on and cook on High for 10 minutes. Release the pressure naturally for 10 minutes, divide everything between plates and serve.

Nutrition: calories 299, fat 14.1, fiber 0.9, carbs 3.9, protein 36.7

Tilapia and Red Sauce

Preparation time: 10 minutes | Cooking time: 20 minutes | Servings: 4

Ingredients:

- 4 tilapia fillets, boneless
- A pinch of salt and black pepper
- 2 tablespoons avocado oil
- 1 tablespoon lemon juice
- 2 spring onions, minced
- ½ cup chicken stock
- ¼ cup tomato passata
- 1 teaspoon garlic powder
- 1 teaspoon oregano, dried
- 1 cup roasted red peppers, chopped
- 10 ounces canned tomatoes and chilies, chopped

Directions:

Set the instant pot on Sauté mode, add the oil, heat it up, add the onions and cook for 2 minutes. Add the rest of the ingredients except the fish and simmer everything for 8 minutes more. Add the fish, put the lid on and cook on High for 10 minutes. Release the pressure naturally for 10 minutes, divide everything between plates and serve.

Nutrition: calories 184, fat 2.2, fiber 1.6, carbs 1.9, protein 22.2

Lime Cod Mix

Preparation time: 10 minutes | Cooking time: 15 minutes | Servings: 4

Ingredients:

- 4 cod fillets, boneless
- ½ teaspoon cumin, ground
- A pinch of salt and black pepper
- 1 tablespoon olive oil
- ½ cup chicken stock
- 3 tablespoons cilantro, chopped
- 2 tablespoons lime juice
- 2 teaspoons lime zest, grated

Directions:

Set the instant pot on Sauté mode, add the oil, heat it up, add the cod and cook for 1 minute on each side. Add the remaining ingredients, put the lid on and cook on High for 13 minutes. Release the pressure naturally for 10 minutes, divide the mix between plates and serve.

Nutrition: calories 187, fat 13.1, fiber 0.2, carbs 1.6, protein 16.1

Salmon and Shrimp Mix

Preparation time: 5 minutes | Cooking time: 20 minutes | Servings: 4

Ingredients:

- 4 salmon fillets, boneless
- 1 pound shrimp, peeled and deveined
- 1 teaspoon Cajun seasoning
- A pinch of salt and black pepper
- 2 tablespoons olive oil
- Juice of 1 lemon
- ½ cup chicken stock
- 2 tablespoons tomato passata

Directions:

Set the instant pot on Sauté mode, add the oil, heat it up, add the rest of the ingredients except the salmon and the shrimp and cook for 3 minutes. Add the salmon and cook for 2 minutes on each side. Add the shrimp, put the lid on and cook on High for 10 minutes. Release the pressure fast for 5 minutes, divide the mix between plates and serve.

Nutrition: calories 393, fat 20, fiber 0.1, carbs 2.2, protein 25

Salmon and Green Beans

Preparation time: 10 minutes | Cooking time: 20 minutes | Servings: 4

Ingredients:

- 4 salmon fillets, boneless
- A pinch of salt and black pepper
- ½ teaspoon sweet paprika
- ½ teaspoon mustard
- ½ teaspoon garlic powder
- 1 tablespoon olive oil
- 1 teaspoon tarragon, dried
- A pinch of salt and black pepper
- ¼ teaspoon dill, chopped
- 1 tablespoons ghee, melted
- ½ cup chicken stock
- 1 pound green beans, trimmed and halved

Directions:

Set the instant pot on Sauté mode, add the oil, heat it up, add the rest of the ingredients except the fish and cook for 5 minutes. Add the fish, put the lid on and cook on High for 15 minutes. Release the pressure naturally for 10 minutes, divide everything between plates and serve.

Nutrition: calories 334, fat 18, fiber 4.3, carbs 5.6, protein 23.7

Cod and Asparagus
Preparation time: 10 minutes | Cooking time: 15 minutes | Servings: 4

Ingredients:
- 4 cod fillets, boneless and skinless
- 2 tablespoons lemon juice
- A pinch of salt and black pepper
- 1 tablespoon parsley, chopped
- 2 tablespoons ghee, melted
- ¼ cup chicken stock
- 1 pound asparagus, trimmed
- ½ teaspoon garlic powder
- 2 teaspoons capers, drained

Directions:
Set the instant pot on Sauté mode, add the ghee, heat it up, add the asparagus and the rest of the ingredients except the fish, and cook for 5 minutes. Add the fish, put the lid on and cook on High for 10 minutes. Release the pressure naturally for 10 minutes, divide everything between plates and serve.

Nutrition: calories 237, fat 16.1, fiber 2.5, carbs 6.2, protein 18.6

Turmeric Shrimp Mix
Preparation time: 5 minutes | Cooking time: 8 minutes | Servings: 4

Ingredients:
- 2 pounds shrimp, peeled and deveined
- A pinch of salt and black pepper
- ½ cup chicken stock
- 1 tablespoon avocado oil
- 1 teaspoon turmeric powder
- 1 tablespoon parsley, chopped

Directions:
Set the instant pot on Sauté mode, add the oil, heat it up, add all the ingredients, toss, put the lid on and cook on High for 8 minutes. Release the pressure fast for 5 minutes, divide the mix between plates and serve.

Nutrition: calories 278, fat 4.4, fiber 0.3, carbs 3.4, protein 27.5

Cod and Basil Tomato Passata

Preparation time: 10 minutes | Cooking time: 12 minutes | Servings: 4

Ingredients:

- 1 pound cod, skinless, boneless and cubed
- 2 tablespoons avocado oil
- 2 garlic cloves, minced
- 10 ounces canned tomatoes, chopped
- 2 tablespoons basil, chopped
- ½ cup veggie stock

Directions:

Set your instant pot on Sauté mode, add the oil, heat it up, add the garlic, stir and brown for 2 minutes. Add the rest of the ingredients, put the lid on and cook on High for 10 minutes. Release the pressure naturally for 10 minutes, divide the mix into bowls and serve.

Nutrition: calories 240, fat 10.7, fiber 1.2, carbs 3.7, protein 31.1

Shrimp and Lemon Green Beans Mix

Preparation time: 10 minutes | Cooking time: 12 minutes | Servings: 4

Ingredients:

- 1 pound shrimp, peeled and deveined
- ½ cup chicken stock
- ½ pound green beans, trimmed and halved
- 1 tablespoon lemon zest, grated
- 1 cup tomato passata
- 1 tablespoon oregano, chopped
- A pinch of salt and black pepper
- 1 tablespoon lemon juice

Directions:

In your instant pot, combine all the ingredients, put the lid on and cook on Low for 12 minutes. Release the pressure naturally for 10 minutes, divide the mix between plates and serve.

Nutrition: calories 174, fat 2.3, fiber 1.2, carbs 1.5, protein 28

Herbed Haddock Mix

Preparation time: 10 minutes | Cooking time: 15 minutes | Servings: 4

Ingredients:

- 2 tablespoons olive oil
- 2 garlic cloves, minced
- ½ cup chicken stock
- 2 tablespoons tomato passata
- A pinch of salt and black pepper
- 1 pound haddock fillets, boneless
- 1 cup red bell pepper, chopped
- ¼ cup tarragon, chopped
- ¼ cup parsley, chopped

Directions:

Set your instant pot on Sauté mode, add the oil, heat it up, add the garlic and the rest of the ingredients except the haddock, stir and cook for 5 minutes. Add the fish, put the lid on and cook on High for 10 minutes. Release the pressure naturally for 10 minutes, divide everything between plates and serve.

Nutrition: calories 209, fat 8.4, fiber 0.8, carbs 4.4, protein 28.6

Salmon and Garlic Spinach

Preparation time: 10 minutes | Cooking time: 15 minutes | Servings: 4

Ingredients:

- 1 and ½ pounds salmon fillets, boneless, skinless
- 1 pound baby spinach
- 3 garlic cloves, minced
- 1 cup tomato passata
- A pinch of salt and black pepper
- 2 tablespoon avocado oil
- 1 tablespoon sage, chopped

Directions:

Set the instant pot on Sauté mode, add the oil, heat it up, add the garlic and the rest of the ingredients except the fish and the spinach, whisk and cook for 5 minutes. Add the fish and the spinach, put the lid on and cook on High for 10 minutes. Release the pressure naturally for 10 minutes, divide everything between plates and serve.

Nutrition: calories 355, fat 15.4, fiber 3.6, carbs 4.6, protein 26.5

Thyme Crab and Spinach

Preparation time: 5 minutes | Cooking time: 14 minutes | Servings: 4

Ingredients:

- 1 tablespoon avocado oil
- 3 cups crab meat
- 1 cup chicken stock
- 2 tablespoons tomato passata
- ½ pound baby spinach
- 1 cup green bell pepper, chopped
- 4 garlic cloves, chopped
- 1 cup tomatoes, cubed
- 2 teaspoons thyme, dried
- A pinch of salt and black pepper

Directions:

Set the instant pot on Sauté mode, add the oil, heat it up, add the garlic, bell pepper and the rest of the ingredients except the crab and the spinach, stir and simmer for 4 minutes. Add the crab and the spinach, put the lid on and cook on High for 10 minutes. Release the pressure fast for 5 minutes, divide the mix between plates and serve.

Nutrition: calories 64, fat 1.4, fiber 0.2, carbs 0.4, protein 5.5

Smoked Crab and Cod Mix

Preparation time: 10 minutes | Cooking time: 12 minutes | Servings: 6

Ingredients:

- 1 pound crab meat
- 1 cup chicken stock
- 1 pound cod fillets, boneless, skinless and cubed
- 2 tablespoons olive oil
- 1 tablespoon smoked paprika
- A pinch of salt and black pepper
- 2 garlic cloves, minced
- 1 tablespoon oregano, chopped
- ½ cup tomato passata

Directions:

Set the instant pot on Sauté mode, add the oil, heat it up, add the garlic and the rest of the ingredients except the cod and the crab, whisk and cook for 5 minutes. Add the crab and the rest of the ingredients, put the lid on and cook on High for 7 minutes. Release the pressure naturally for 10 minutes, divide the mix between plates and serve.

Nutrition: calories 300, fat 15.7, fiber 1.6, carbs 3.5, protein 21.5

Rosemary Tilapia and Pine Nuts

Preparation time: 10 minutes | Cooking time: 15 minutes | Servings: 4

Ingredients:

- 4 tilapia fillets, skinless and boneless
- ¼ cup avocado oil
- Juice of 1 lime
- 1 tablespoon lime zest, grated
- 4 garlic cloves, minced
- ½ cup pine nuts
- 1 tablespoon rosemary, chopped
- A pinch of salt and black pepper
- 1 cup chicken stock
- 1 teaspoon sweet paprika

Directions:

Set the instant pot on Sauté mode, add the oil, heat it up, add the garlic and the rest of the ingredients except the fish, whisk and cook for 5 minutes. Add the fish, put the lid on and cook on High for 10 minutes. Release the pressure naturally for 10 minutes, divide the mix between plates and serve.

Nutrition: calories 170, fat 14, fiber 2, carbs 5.3, protein 8.3

Crab, Spinach and Chives

Preparation time: 10 minutes | Cooking time: 10 minutes | Servings: 4

Ingredients:

- 1 pound crab meat
- 1 cup baby spinach
- 1 cup chicken stock
- ¼ cup tomato passata
- 1 tablespoon olive oil
- 1 tablespoon chives, chopped

Directions:

In your instant pot, combine the crab meat with the spinach and the rest of the ingredients, put the lid on and cook on High for 10 minutes. Release the pressure naturally for 10 minutes, divide the mix between plates and serve.

Nutrition: calories 139, fat 5.7, fiber 0.4, carbs 3.3, protein 14.2

Chili Haddock and Tomatoes
Preparation time: 10 minutes | Cooking time: 15 minutes | Servings: 4

Ingredients:
- 4 haddock fillets, boneless
- 1 tablespoon red chili powder
- A pinch of salt and black pepper
- ½ cup chicken stock
- 1 cup tomatoes, cubed
- 4 garlic cloves, minced
- 2 tablespoons avocado oil
- 1 tablespoon chives, chopped

Directions:
Set the instant pot on Sauté mode, add the oil, heat it up, add the garlic and the rest of the ingredients except the fish and the chives, whisk and cook for 5 minutes. Add the fish, put the lid on and cook on High for 10 minutes. Release the pressure naturally for 10 minutes, divide the mix into bowls and serve with the chives sprinkled on top.

Nutrition: calories 197, fat 2.8, fiber 1.5, carbs 2.2, protein 26.4

Tuna and Green Beans Mix
Preparation time: 10 minutes | Cooking time: 12 minutes | Servings: 4

Ingredients:
- 1 pound tuna, skinless, boneless and cubed
- 1 pound green beans, trimmed
- 1 and ½ cups tomato passata
- 1 tablespoons olive oil
- ½ teaspoon sweet paprika
- 1 teaspoon oregano, dried
- Salt and black pepper to the taste

Directions:
Set your instant pot on Sauté mode, add the oil, heat it up, add the green beans and the rest of the ingredients except the tuna, stir and cook for 5 minutes. Add the tuna, put the lid on and cook on High for 7 minutes. Release the pressure naturally for 10 minutes, divide the mix into bowls and serve.

Nutrition: calories 278, fat 12.7, fiber 3.6, carbs 4.5, protein 27.5

Chipotle Tilapia Mix

Preparation time: 10 minutes | Cooking time: 15 minutes | Servings: 4

Ingredients:

- 4 tilapia fillets, boneless
- 2 garlic cloves, minced
- 1 teaspoon chipotle chili powder
- 2 spring onions, chopped
- ½ tablespoon lime juice
- A pinch of salt and black pepper
- 1 tablespoon olive oil
- 1 cup chicken stock
- 1 tablespoon parsley, chopped
- 2 tablespoons tomato passata

Directions:

Set your instant pot on Sauté mode, add the oil, heat it up, add the garlic, chili powder and the rest of the ingredients except the tilapia and the parsley, stir and cook for 5 minutes. Add the fish, put the lid on and cook on High for 10 minutes. Release the pressure naturally for 10 minutes, divide the mix between plates and serve with the parsley sprinkled on top.

Nutrition: calories 250, fat 14.9, fiber 0.4, carbs 5.5, protein 13.9

Ginger Halibut

Preparation time: 10 minutes | Cooking time: 15 minutes | Servings: 4

Ingredients:

- 4 halibut fillets, boneless
- 1 cup tomatoes, chopped
- 1 tablespoon ginger, grated
- ¼ cup chicken stock
- 1 tablespoon sweet paprika
- 1 tablespoon chives, chopped

Directions:

Set the instant pot on Sauté mode, add the ginger and the rest of the ingredients except the fish, toss and cook for 3 minutes. Add the fish, put the lid on and cook on High for 12 minutes. Release the pressure naturally for 10 minutes, divide the mix between plates and serve.

Nutrition: calories 337, fat 7.1, fiber 1.4, carbs 3.8, protein 18.6

Halibut and Brussels Sprouts
Preparation time: 5 minutes | Cooking time: 12 minutes | Servings: 4

Ingredients:
- 4 halibut fillets, boneless and skinless
- 1 pound Brussels sprouts, halved
- 2 garlic cloves, minced
- 1 tablespoon avocado oil
- 1 cup tomato passata
- A pinch of salt and black pepper
- 1 tablespoon parsley, chopped

Directions:
Set the instant pot on Sauté mode, add the oil, heat it up, add the garlic and cook for 2 minutes Add the rest of the ingredients, put the lid on and cook on High for 10 minutes. Release the pressure fast for 5 minutes, divide everything between plates and serve.

Nutrition: calories 389, fat 7.7, fiber 5.4, carbs 6.1, protein 18.7

Creamy Catfish
Preparation time: 10 minutes | Cooking time: 12 minutes | Servings: 4

Ingredients:
- 1 pound catfish fillets, boneless, skinless and cubed
- 1 and ½ cups coconut milk
- 2 garlic cloves, minced
- 1 tablespoon ginger, grated
- ½ teaspoon yellow curry paste
- A pinch of salt and black pepper
- 2 tablespoons lime juice
- 1 tablespoon parsley, chopped

Directions:
In your instant pot, mix the fish with the coconut milk and the rest of the ingredients except the parsley, put the lid on and cook on High for 12 minutes. Release the pressure naturally for 10 minutes, divide everything into bowls and serve.

Nutrition: calories 274, fat 14.4, fiber 0.9, carbs 4.5, protein 16.9

Ketogenic Instant Pot Poultry Recipes

Oregano Chicken
Preparation time: 10 minutes | Cooking time: 20 minutes | Servings: 4

Ingredients:

- 2 chicken breasts, skinless, boneless and cubed
- 1 cup tomato passata
- ½ cup chicken stock
- 1 tablespoon oregano, chopped
- A pinch of salt and black pepper
- 1 teaspoon sweet paprika
- 1 tablespoon cilantro, chopped

Directions:

In your instant pot, combine all the ingredients, toss, put the lid on and cook on High for 20 minutes. Release the pressure naturally for 10 minutes, divide the mix between plates and serve.

Nutrition: calories 183, fat 2.5, fiber 1.2, carbs 1.5, protein 13.4

Spiced Chicken Bites
Preparation time: 10 minutes | Cooking time: 24 minutes | Servings: 4

Ingredients:

- 2 chicken breasts, skinless, boneless and cubed
- 2 tablespoons avocado oil
- ½ teaspoon turmeric powder
- ½ teaspoon cumin, ground
- ½ teaspoon allspice, ground
- ½ teaspoon cinnamon powder
- 1 teaspoon sweet paprika
- 2 tablespoons tomato paste
- 1 cup chicken stock

Directions:

Set your instant pot on Sauté mode, add the oil, heat it up, add the chicken and brown for 2 minutes on each side. Add the rest of the ingredients, put the lid on and cook on High for 20 minutes Release the pressure naturally for 10 minutes, divide the mix between plates and serve.

Nutrition: calories 238, fat 9.7, fiber 1, carbs 2.9, protein 33.3

Coconut Chicken and Peppers

Preparation time: 10 minutes | Cooking time: 24 minutes | Servings: 4

Ingredients:

- 1 cup chicken stock
- A pinch of salt and black pepper
- 1 pound chicken breast, skinless, boneless and cubed
- 1 tablespoon coconut, unsweetened and shredded
- 1 tablespoon oregano, chopped
- ½ pound mixed peppers, cut into strips
- 1 tablespoon chives, chopped
- 1 tablespoon olive oil

Directions:

Set your instant pot on Sauté mode, add the oil, heat it up, add the onion and the chicken and brown for 2 minutes on each side. Add the rest of the ingredients, put the lid on and cook on High for 20 minutes. Release the pressure naturally for 10 minutes, divide everything between plates and serve.

Nutrition: calories 256, fat 12.6, fiber 0.6, carbs 1.2, protein 33.2

Basil Chili Chicken

Preparation time: 5 minutes | Cooking time: 24 minutes | Servings: 4

Ingredients:

- 1 pound chicken breast, skinless, boneless and cubed
- A pinch of salt and black pepper
- 1 tablespoon chili powder
- 1 cup coconut cream
- 2 teaspoons sweet paprika
- ½ cup chicken stock
- 2 tablespoons basil, chopped

Directions:

In your instant pot, combine the chicken with the rest of the ingredients,   toss a bit, put the lid on and cook on High for 24 minutes. Release the pressure naturally for 10 minutes, divide the mix between plates and serve.

Nutrition: calories 364, fat 23.2, fiber 2.3, carbs 5.1, protein 35.4

Chicken and Oregano Sauce

Preparation time: 10 minutes | Cooking time: 20 minutes | Servings: 4

Ingredients:

- 2 chicken breasts, skinless, boneless and halved
- 1 tablespoon lemon juice
- 2 tablespoons olive oil
- 2 tablespoons oregano, chopped
- 1 cup tomato passata
- 1 teaspoon ginger, grated

Directions:

Set the instant pot on Sauté mode, add the oil, heat it up, add tomato passata and the rest of the ingredients except the chicken, whisk and cook for 5 minutes. Add the chicken, put the lid on and cook on High for 15 minutes. Release the pressure naturally for 10 minutes, divide the mix between plates and serve.

Nutrition: calories 300, fat 15.8, fiber 2, carbs 5.2, protein 33.9

Balsamic Curry Chicken

Preparation time: 10 minutes | Cooking time: 20 minutes | Servings: 4

Ingredients:

- 1 pound chicken breast, skinless, boneless and cubed
- A pinch of salt and black pepper
- 1 cup chicken stock
- 1 cup coconut cream
- 3 garlic cloves, minced
- 1 and ½ tablespoon balsamic vinegar
- 1 tablespoon chives, chopped

Directions:

In your instant pot, combine the chicken with the rest of the ingredients, put the lid on and cook on High for 20 minutes. Release the pressure naturally for 10 minutes, divide the mix between plates and serve.

Nutrition: calories 360, fat 22.1, fiber 1.4, carbs 4.3, protein 34.5

Chicken and Eggplant Mix

Preparation time: 10 minutes | Cooking time: 20 minutes | Servings: 4

Ingredients:

- 2 chicken breasts, skinless, boneless and halved
- A pinch of salt and black pepper
- 2 eggplants, roughly cubed
- 2 tablespoons olive oil
- 1 cup tomato passata
- 1 tablespoon oregano, dried

Directions:

In your instant pot, combine all the ingredients, put the lid on and cook on High for 20 minutes. Release the pressure naturally for 10 minutes, divide between plates and serve.

Nutrition: calories 362, fat 16.1, fiber 4.4, carbs 5.4, protein 36.4

Sesame Chicken

Preparation time: 10 minutes | Cooking time: 20 minutes | Servings: 4

Ingredients:

- 2 chicken breasts, skinless, boneless and cubed
- A pinch of salt and black pepper
- 1 teaspoon sesame seeds
- 4 garlic cloves, minced
- 1 cup tomato passata
- 1 tablespoon parsley, chopped
- 1 tablespoon oregano, chopped

Directions:

In your instant pot, mix all the ingredients except the sesame seeds, put the lid on and cook on High for 20 minutes. Release the pressure naturally for 10 minutes, divide everything between plates and serve with the sesame seeds sprinkled on top.

Nutrition: calories 243, fat 9, fiber 1.6, carbs 5.4, protein 34.1

Turkey and Spring Onions Mix

Preparation time: 10 minutes | Cooking time: 25 minutes | Servings: 4

Ingredients:

- 1 turkey breast, skinless, boneless and cubed
- 2 tablespoons avocado oil
- 4 spring onions, chopped
- 1 cup tomato passata
- A handful cilantro, chopped
- A pinch of salt and black pepper

Directions:

Set your instant pot on Sauté mode, add the oil, heat it up, add the meat and brown for 5 minutes. Add the rest of the ingredients, put the lid on and cook on High for 20 minutes. Release the pressure naturally for 10 minutes between plates, divide the turkey mix between plates, and serve.

Nutrition: calories 222, fat 6.7, fiber 1.6, carbs 4.8, protein 34.4

Italian Paprika Chicken

Preparation time: 10 minutes | Cooking time: 20 minutes | Servings: 4

Ingredients:

- 1 pound chicken breasts, skinless, boneless and cubed
- A pinch of salt and black pepper
- 1 tablespoon olive oil
- 1 tablespoon sweet paprika
- 1 tablespoon Italian seasoning
- 2 garlic cloves, minced
- 1 and ½ cups chicken stock

Directions:

Set your instant pot on Sauté mode, add the oil, heat it up, add the meat and brown for 5 minutes. Add the rest of the ingredients, put the lid on and cook on High for 15 minutes. Release the pressure naturally for 10 minutes, divide between plates and serve.

Nutrition: calories 264, fat 13.2, fiber 0.7, carbs 1.9, protein 33.2

Tomato Turkey and Sprouts

Preparation time: 10 minutes | Cooking time: 25 minutes | Servings: 4

Ingredients:

- 1 big turkey breast, skinless, boneless and cubed
- 1 tablespoon avocado oil
- 1 pound Brussels sprouts
- 1 teaspoon chili powder
- 1 and ½ cups tomato passata
- 2 tablespoons cilantro, chopped
- A pinch of salt and black pepper

Directions:

Set the instant pot on Sauté mode, add the oil, heat it up, add the meat and brown for 5 minutes. Add the rest of the ingredients, put the lid on and cook on High for 20 minutes. Release the pressure naturally for 10 minutes, divide the mix between plates and serve.

Nutrition: calories 249, fat 6.6, fiber 2.5, carbs 4.5, protein 37.3

Chicken, Kale and Artichokes

Preparation time: 10 minutes | Cooking time: 25 minutes | Servings: 4

Ingredients:

- 1 pound chicken breast, skinless, boneless and cubed
- 1 shallot, minced
- 4 garlic cloves, minced
- 1 pound kale, torn
- A pinch of salt and black pepper
- 1 cup canned artichoke hearts, drained
- 1 cup chicken stock
- 2 tablespoons avocado oil

Directions:

Set your instant pot on Sauté mode, add the oil, heat it up, add the shallot, garlic and the chicken and sauté for 5 minutes. Add the rest of the ingredients, toss, put the lid on and cook on High for 20 minutes. Release the pressure naturally for 10 minutes, divide the mix between plates and serve.

Nutrition: calories 288, fat 9.5, fiber 2.1, carbs 5.6, protein 38.6

Sage Chicken and Broccoli

Preparation time: 10 minutes | Cooking time: 30 minutes | Servings: 4

Ingredients:

- 1 pound chicken breast, skinless, boneless and cubed
- 1 cup broccoli florets
- 3 garlic cloves, minced
- 1 cup tomato passata
- A pinch of salt and black pepper
- 2 tablespoons olive oil
- 1 tablespoon sage, chopped

Directions:

Set pot on Sauté mode, add the oil, heat it up, add the garlic and the chicken and sauté for 5 minutes. Add the rest of the ingredients, put the lid on and cook on High for 25 minutes. Release the pressure naturally for 10 minutes, divide the mix between plates and serve.

Nutrition: calories 217, fat 10.1, fiber 1.8, carbs 5.9, protein 25.4

Turkey and Cabbage Mix

Preparation time: 10 minutes | Cooking time: 30 minutes | Servings: 4

Ingredients:

- 2 turkey breasts, skinless, boneless and cubed
- 1 red cabbage, shredded
- 1 cup chicken stock
- 2 tablespoons tomato puree
- ½ teaspoon chili powder
- A pinch of salt and black pepper

Directions:

In your instant pot, combine the turkey meat with the rest of the ingredients, put the lid on and cook on High for 30 minutes. Release the pressure naturally for 10 minutes, divide everything between plates and serve.

Nutrition: calories 392, fat 11.6, fiber 0.3, carbs 1.1, protein 24.2

Balsamic Turkey and Zucchini

Preparation time: 10 minutes | Cooking time: 25 minutes | Servings: 4

Ingredients:
- 1 big turkey breast, skinless, boneless and cubed
- 1 and ½ cups chicken stock
- A pinch of salt and black pepper
- 2 zucchinis, sliced
- 3 garlic cloves, minced
- 1 tablespoon balsamic vinegar
- 1 tablespoon olive oil
- 1 tablespoon chili powder
- ½ teaspoon sweet paprika

Directions:
Set the instant pot on Sauté mode, add the oil, heat it up, add the garlic, chili powder, paprika and the meat and brown for 5 minutes. Add the rest of the ingredients, put the lid on and cook on High for 20 minutes. Release the pressure naturally for 10 minutes, divide the mix between plates and serve.

Nutrition: calories 249, fat 9.7, fiber 1.9, carbs 5.3, protein 34.3

Ginger Balsamic Chicken

Preparation time: 10 minutes | Cooking time: 25 minutes | Servings: 4

Ingredients:
- 2 chicken breasts, skinless, boneless and cubed
- 2 spring onions, chopped
- 1 tablespoon balsamic vinegar
- 1 tablespoon ginger, grated
- 1 tablespoon olive oil
- 3 garlic cloves, minced
- A pinch of salt and black pepper
- 1 cup chicken stock
- 2 tablespoons sweet paprika
- 1 tablespoon cilantro, chopped

Directions:
Set the instant pot on Sauté mode, add the oil, heat it up, add the spring onions, ginger, garlic and the meat and brown for 5 minutes. Add the rest of the ingredients, put the lid on and cook on High for 20 minutes. Release the pressure naturally for 10 minutes, divide the mix between plates and serve.

Nutrition: calories 269, fat 12.6, fiber 1.7, carbs 4.4, protein 33.9

Tarragon Chicken Mix

Preparation time: 5 minutes | Cooking time: 25 minutes | Servings: 4

Ingredients:

- 2 chicken breasts, skinless and halved
- 1 shallot, chopped
- 1 and ½ teaspoon tarragon, dried
- 1 cup tomato passata
- A pinch of salt and black pepper
- 1 cup tomatoes, cubed
- ½ cup red cabbage, shredded

Directions:

In your instant pot, mix the chicken with the rest of the ingredients, put the lid on and cook on High for 25 minutes. Release the pressure fast for 5 minutes, divide the mix between plates and serve.

Nutrition: calories 241, fat 8.6, fiber 1.5, carbs 5.6, protein 34.1

Duck and Fennel

Preparation time: 10 minutes | Cooking time: 25 minutes | Servings: 4

Ingredients:

- 2 duck breasts, boneless and skin scored
- 1 cup chicken stock
- 2 fennel bulbs, sliced
- Juice of 1 lime
- 1 tablespoon avocado oil
- 1 cup tomato passata
- 1 tablespoon parsley, chopped

Directions:

Set the instant pot on Sauté mode, add the oil, heat it up, add the duck breasts skin side down and cook for 5 minutes. Add the rest of the ingredients except the parsley, put the lid on and cook on High for 20 minutes. Release the pressure naturally for 10 minutes, divide the mix between plates and serve with the parsley sprinkled on top.

Nutrition: calories 260, fat 7.7, fiber 3.4, carbs 4.5, protein 34.5

Chicken and Herbs Sauce

Preparation time: 10 minutes | Cooking time: 25 minutes | Servings: 4

Ingredients:

- 2 chicken breasts, skinless, boneless and halved
- 2 tablespoons ghee, melted
- 1 cup chicken stock
- 2 bay leaves
- A pinch of salt and black pepper
- 1 tablespoon chervil, chopped
- 1 tablespoon chives, chopped
- 1 tablespoon cilantro, chopped
- 1 tablespoon thyme, chopped

Directions:

Set your instant pot on Sauté mode, add the ghee, heat it up, add the chervil, chives, cilantro, bay leaves and thyme and cook for 2 minutes. Add the meat and brown for 3 minutes more. Add the rest of the ingredients, put the lid on and cook on High for 20 minutes. Release the pressure naturally for 10 minutes, divide the mix between plates and serve.

Nutrition: calories 277, fat 15, fiber 0.3, carbs 0.9, protein 33.2

Turkey and Lime Dill Sauce

Preparation time: 5 minutes | Cooking time: 30 minutes | Servings: 4

Ingredients:

- 1 big turkey breast, skinless, boneless and cubed
- 1 tablespoon ghee, melted
- 1 and ½ tablespoons lime zest, grated
- 1 tablespoon lime juice
- 1 cup chicken stock
- 1 tablespoon dill, chopped
- 1 tablespoon smoked paprika
- A pinch of salt and black pepper

Directions:

Set the instant pot on Sauté mode, add the ghee, heat it up, add lime zest, juice, stock, dill and paprika, whisk and cook for 5 minutes. Add the meat, salt and pepper, put the lid on and cook on High for 25 minutes. Release the pressure fast for 5 minutes, divide the mix between plates and serve.

Nutrition: calories 230, fat 9.2, fiber 0.8, carbs 1.6, protein 33.8

Hot Curry Turkey

Preparation time: 5 minutes | Cooking time: 30 minutes | Servings: 4

Ingredients:

- 1 big turkey breast, skinless, boneless and cubed
- 2 curry leaves
- 1 tablespoon green curry paste
- 4 tablespoons hot sauce
- 1 cup chicken stock
- 2 tablespoons tomato passata
- 1 tablespoon chives, chopped

Directions:

In your instant pot, combine the turkey with the rest of the ingredients, put the lid on and cook on High for 30 minutes. Release the pressure fast for 5 minutes, discard curry leaves, divide the mix into bowls and serve.

Nutrition: calories 210, fat 6.6, fiber 0.2, carbs 2, protein 33.6

Duck and Hot Eggplant Mix

Preparation time: 10 minutes | Cooking time: 30 minutes | Servings: 4

Ingredients:

- 2 duck legs, skinless, boneless and cubed
- 1 tablespoon olive oil
- 2 eggplants, sliced
- A pinch of salt and black pepper
- 1 tablespoon hot paprika
- 2 tablespoons tomato paste
- 2 cups chicken stock
- 1 and ½ teaspoons chili powder
- 1 tablespoon cilantro, chopped

Directions:

Set your instant pot on Sauté mode, add the oil, heat it up, add the meat and the rest of the ingredients except the eggplants, stock and cilantro, toss and cook for 5 minutes. Add the eggplant and stock, put the lid on and cook on High for 25 minutes. Release the pressure naturally for 10 minutes, divide the mix between plates and serve with the cilantro sprinkled on top.

Nutrition: calories 338, fat 17, fiber 2.6, carbs 6.6, protein 30

Chicken, Cabbage and Leeks

Preparation time: 10 minutes | Cooking time: 30 minutes | Servings: 4

Ingredients:

- 2 chicken breasts, skinless, boneless and cubed
- A pinch of salt and black pepper
- 1 tablespoon ghee, melted
- 1 red cabbage, shredded
- 2 leeks, sliced
- 1 cup chicken stock
- 1 tablespoon tomato passata
- 1 tablespoon basil, chopped
- 1 tablespoon balsamic vinegar

Directions:

Set the instant pot on Sauté mode, add the ghee, heat it up, add the meat and the leeks and brown for 5 minutes. Add the rest of the ingredients except the basil, toss, put the lid on and cook on High for 25 minutes Release the pressure naturally for 10 minutes, divide the mix between plates, sprinkle the basil on top and serve.

Nutrition: calories 275, fat 11.9, fiber 0.6, carbs 6.7, protein 33.7

Turkey and Spicy Okra

Preparation time: 10 minutes | Cooking time: 30 minutes | Servings: 4

Ingredients:

- 2 cups okra, trimmed
- 1 shallot, chopped
- 1 tablespoon olive oil
- 2 garlic cloves, minced
- 1 turkey breast, skinless, boneless and cubed
- 1 tablespoon chili powder
- 1 cup tomato passata
- A pinch of salt and black pepper
- 1 tablespoon parsley, chopped
- 1 tablespoon oregano, chopped

Directions:

Set the instant pot on Sauté mode, add the oil, heat it up, add the shallot, garlic, turkey and the chili powder and brown for 5 minutes. Add the rest of the ingredients except the parsley and the oregano, put the lid on and cook on High for 25 minutes. Release the pressure naturally for 10 minutes, divide the mix between plates, sprinkle the parsley and oregano on top and serve.

Nutrition: calories 279, fat 9.8, fiber 3.5, carbs 5.6, protein 35.4

Chicken and Balsamic Mushrooms

Preparation time: 10 minutes | Cooking time: 20 minutes | Servings: 4

Ingredients:

- 2 chicken breasts, skinless, boneless and cubed
- 1 tablespoon balsamic vinegar
- 1 pound white mushrooms, sliced
- 1 tablespoon rosemary, chopped
- 1 cup chicken stock
- A pinch of salt and black pepper
- 1 tablespoon avocado oil
- 2 tablespoons tomato passata

Directions:

Set your instant pot on Sauté mode, add the oil, heat it up, add the chicken and the mushrooms and brown for 5 minutes. Add the rest of the ingredients, put the lid on and cook on High for 20 minutes. Release the pressure naturally for 10 minutes, divide everything between plates and serve.

Nutrition: calories 252, fat 9.4, fiber 1.8, carbs 5.1, protein 36.4

Creamy Turkey and Chard

Preparation time: 10 minutes | Cooking time: 30 minutes | Servings: 4

Ingredients:

- 1 turkey breast, skinless, boneless and cubed
- 1 tablespoon ghee, melted
- 2 garlic cloves, minced
- 1 and ½ cup coconut cream
- 1 cup chard, roughly chopped
- ½ bunch coriander, chopped

Directions:

Set your instant pot on Sauté mode, add the ghee, heat it up, add the meat and the garlic and brown for 5 minutes. Add the rest of the ingredients, put the lid on and cook on High for 25 minutes. Release the pressure naturally for 10 minutes, divide the mix between plates and serve.

Nutrition: calories 225, fat 8.9, fiber 0.2, carbs 0.8, protein 33.5

Duck and Coriander Sauce
Preparation time: 10 minutes | Cooking time: 30 minutes | Servings: 4

Ingredients:
- 1 pound duck legs, boneless, skinless and cubed
- 2 tablespoons ghee, melt
- 2 spring onions, chopped
- 2 garlic cloves, minced
- 1 and ½ cups tomato passata
- 2 tablespoon coriander, chopped

Directions:
Set your instant pot on Sauté mode, add the ghee, heat it up, add the spring onions and the rest of the ingredients except the meat and the tomato passata and brown for 5 minutes. Add the meat and brown for 5 minutes more. Add the sauce, put the lid on and cook on High for 25 minutes. Release the pressure naturally for 10 minutes, divide between plates and serve.

Nutrition: calories 263, fat 13.2, fiber 0.2, carbs 1.1, protein 33.5

Chicken, Baby Kale and Spinach Mix
Preparation time: 5 minutes | Cooking time: 30 minutes | Servings: 4

Ingredients:
- 1 tablespoon ghee, melted
- 1 pound chicken breasts, skinless, boneless and cubed
- 1 pound baby kale
- ½ pound baby spinach
- 1 cup tomato passata
- A pinch of salt and black pepper
- 1 cup chicken stock
- 1 tablespoon chives, chopped

Directions:
Set your instant pot on Sauté mode, add the ghee, heat it up, add the meat and brown for 5 minutes. Add the rest of the ingredients except the kale and the spinach, put the lid on and cook on High for 15 minutes. Release the pressure fast for 5 minutes, set the pot on Sauté mode, add the kale and spinach, cook for 10 minutes more, divide between plates and serve.

Nutrition: calories 274, fat 12.1, fiber 2.2, carbs 5.6, protein 35.4

Chicken and Cauliflower Rice

Preparation time: 5 minutes | Cooking time: 30 minutes | Servings: 6

Ingredients:

- 1 and ½ pounds chicken breasts, skinless, boneless and cubed
- 1 and ½ cups cauliflower rice
- 2 tablespoons ghee, melted
- 1 tablespoon sweet paprika
- ½ teaspoon chili powder
- 2 cups chicken stock
- 1 tablespoon cilantro, chopped
- A pinch of salt and black pepper

Directions:

Set the instant pot on Sauté mode, add the ghee, heat it up, add the meat, paprika and chili powder and brown for 5 minutes. Add the rest of the ingredients, put the lid on and cook on High for 25 minutes. Release the pressure fast for 5 minutes, divide everything between plates and serve.

Nutrition: calories 332, fat 15.4, fiber 0.5, carbs 1, protein 34.5

Turkey and Mustard Greens Mix

Preparation time: 10 minutes | Cooking time: 30 minutes | Servings: 6

Ingredients:

- 2 turkey breasts, skinless, boneless and cubed
- 1 tablespoon olive oil
- 2 garlic cloves, minced
- 1 cup chicken stock
- 1 and ½ cup tomato passata
- 1 pound mustard greens, torn
- 1 tablespoon smoked paprika
- 1 tablespoon cilantro, chopped
- A pinch of salt and black pepper

Directions:

Set the instant pot on Sauté mode, add the oil, heat it up, add the meat, garlic and paprika and brown for 5 minutes. Add the rest of the ingredients except the cilantro, put the lid on and cook on High for 25 minutes. Release the pressure naturally for 10 minutes, divide the mix between plates and serve with the cilantro sprinkled on top.

Nutrition: calories 262, fat 9.8, fiber 4.2, carbs 5.8, protein 34.6

Turkey and Rocket Mix

Preparation time: 5 minutes | Cooking time: 30 minutes | Servings: 4

Ingredients:

- 1 turkey breast, skinless, boneless and sliced
- ½ cup chicken stock
- 2 tablespoons tomato passata
- 1 shallot, minced
- 2 garlic cloves, minced
- 1 cup rocket leaves
- 1 tablespoon avocado oil
- ¼ cup cilantro, chopped

Directions:

Set the instant pot on Sauté mode, add the oil, heat it up, add the meat, shallot and the garlic and brown for 5 minutes Add the remaining ingredients except the cilantro and the rocket, put the lid on and cook on High for 25 minutes. Release the pressure fast for 5 minutes, divide everything between plates and serve with the cilantro and rocket sprinkled on top.

Nutrition: calories 204, fat 6.2, fiber 0,4, carbs 1.6, protein 33.4

Chicken and Watercress Mix

Preparation time: 5 minutes | Cooking time: 30 minutes | Servings: 4

Ingredients:

- 2 chicken breasts, skinless, boneless and halved
- 2 spring onions, chopped
- 2 garlic cloves, minced
- 1 tablespoon olive oil
- 1 cup chicken stock
- ½ cup tomato passata
- A pinch of salt and black pepper
- 1 cup watercress, torn

Directions:

Set the instant pot on Sauté mode, add the oil, heat it up, add the spring onions, garlic and the meat and brown for 5 minutes. Add the rest of the ingredients except the watercress, put the lid on and cook on High for 25 minutes. Release the pressure fast for 5 minutes, divide the mix between plates and serve with the watercress on top.

Nutrition: calories 262, fat 12.2, fiber 0.8, carbs 2.9, protein 33.8

Duck, Leeks and Asparagus

Preparation time: 10 minutes | Cooking time: 30 minutes | Servings: 4

Ingredients:

- 2 tablespoons ghee, melted
- 2 duck legs, boneless, skinless and cubed
- 1 shallot, chopped
- 2 leeks, sliced
- ½ pound asparagus, trimmed and halved
- 1 cup chicken stock
- A pinch of salt and black pepper
- 2 teaspoons basil, dried
- 1 teaspoon oregano, dried

Directions:

Set your instant pot on Sauté mode, add the ghee, heat it up, add the shallot, leeks and the meat and brown for 5 minutes. Add the rest of the ingredients, put the lid on and cook on High for 25 minutes. Release the pressure naturally for 10 minutes, divide the mix between plates and serve.

Nutrition: calories 300, fat 13.5, fiber 2.2, carbs 6.7, protein 35.2

Chicken and Garlic Spinach

Preparation time: 10 minutes | Cooking time: 25 minutes | Servings: 4

Ingredients:

- 3 garlic cloves, minced
- 2 tablespoons ghee, melted
- 1 pound baby spinach
- 1 pound chicken breasts, skinless, boneless and cubed
- A pinch of salt and black pepper
- 1 cup chicken stock
- 2 tablespoons cilantro, chopped

Directions:

Set your instant pot on Sauté mode, add the ghee, heat it up, add the garlic and the meat and brown for 5 minutes. Add the rest of the ingredients except the spinach, put the lid on and cook on High for 15 minutes. Release the pressure naturally for 10 minutes, set the pot on Sauté mode again, add the spinach, cook for 5 minutes more, divide everything between plates and serve.

Nutrition: calories 304, fat 15.4, fiber 2.6, carbs 5.1, protein 36.

Turmeric Duck Mix

*Preparation time: 5 minutes | **Cooking time:** 30 minutes | Servings: 4*

Ingredients:

- 1 shallot, chopped
- 1 tablespoon olive oil
- 2 garlic cloves, minced
- 1 pound duck legs, boneless, skinless and cubed
- 1 cup chicken stock
- 1 tablespoon cilantro, chopped
- 1 teaspoon turmeric powder
- A pinch of salt and black pepper

Directions:

Set your instant pot on Sauté mode, add the oil, heat it up, add the shallot, garlic and the meat and brown for 5 minutes. Add the rest of the ingredients except the cilantro, put the lid on and cook on High for 25 minutes. Release the pressure fast for 5 minutes, divide the mix between plates and serve with the cilantro sprinkled on top.

Nutrition: calories 239, fat 10.5, fiber 0.2, carbs 1.1, protein 33.3

Turkey and Hot Lemon Sauce

*Preparation time: 10 minutes | **Cooking time:** 30 minutes | Servings: 4*

Ingredients:

- 2 turkey breasts, skinless, boneless and cubed
- 1 shallot, minced
- 1 tablespoon ghee, melted
- 1 tablespoon lemon juice
- 1 tablespoon lemon zest, grated
- A pinch of salt and black pepper
- 1 teaspoon red pepper flakes
- 1 cup chicken stock

Directions:

Set your instant pot on Sauté mode, add the ghee, heat it up, add the shallot and the meat and brown for 5 minutes. Add the rest of the ingredients, put the lid on and cook on High for 25 minutes. Release the pressure naturally for 10 minutes, divide everything between plates and serve.

Nutrition: calories 227, fat 9.1, fiber 0.2, carbs 0.8, protein 33.5

Oregano Chicken and Dates

Preparation time: 10 minutes | Cooking time: 25 minutes | Servings: 4

Ingredients:

- 1 pound chicken breast, skinless, boneless and cubed
- 1 tablespoon olive oil
- 1 tablespoon oregano, chopped
- 1 cup chicken stock
- 1 cup dates, pitted and chopped
- 1 tablespoon chives, chopped
- 1 tablespoon sweet paprika
- A pinch of salt and black pepper

Directions:

Set your instant pot on Sauté mode, add the oil, heat it up, add the meat and brown for 5 minutes. Add the rest of the ingredients, put the lid on and cook on High for 20 minutes. Release the pressure naturally for 10 minutes, divide everything between plates and serve.

Nutrition: calories 382, fat 12.6, fiber 2.6, carbs 6.6, protein 33.6

White Duck Chili

Preparation time: 10 minutes | Cooking time: 25 minutes | Servings: 4

Ingredients:

- 2 duck legs, boneless, skinless and cubed
- 1 tablespoon ghee, melted
- 1 shallot, chopped
- 1 cup heavy cream
- 1 and ½ teaspoons chili paste
- 1 cup chicken stock
- A pinch of salt and black pepper
- 2 teaspoons thyme, dried

Directions:

Set the instant pot on Sauté mode, add the ghee, heat it up, add the shallot and the meat and brown for 5 minutes. Add the rest of the ingredients, put the lid on and cook on High for 25 minutes. Release the pressure naturally for 10 minutes, divide everything into bowls and serve.

Nutrition: calories 337, fat 21.2, fiber 0.2, carbs 1.4, protein 33.6

Chicken, Radish and Green Beans

Preparation time: 10 minutes | Cooking time: 25 minutes | Servings: 4

Ingredients:

- 2 chicken breasts, skinless, boneless and cubed
- 1 cup radishes, sliced
- 1 pound green beans, trimmed and halved
- 1 and ½ cups chicken stock
- 1 tablespoon tomato passata
- A pinch of salt and black pepper
- 1 teaspoon chili powder
- 1 tablespoon chives, chopped

Directions:

In your instant pot, mix chicken with the radishes and the rest of the ingredients except the chives, put the lid on and cook on High for 25 minutes. Release the pressure naturally for 10 minutes, divide everything between plates and serve.

Nutrition: calories 259, fat 8.7, fiber 4.3, carbs 6.5, protein 35.4

Cinnamon Turkey and Celery Mix

Preparation time: 10 minutes | Cooking time: 20 minutes | Servings: 4

Ingredients:

- 1 turkey breast, skinless, boneless and cubed
- 1 tablespoon sweet paprika
- 1 tablespoon tomato passata
- 1 cup chicken stock
- 1 tablespoon ghee, melted
- 2 celery stalks, chopped
- A pinch of salt and black pepper
- ½ teaspoon cinnamon powder
- 1 tablespoon cilantro, chopped

Directions:

Set instant pot on Sauté mode, add the ghee, heat it up, add the meat and the cinnamon and brown for 5 minutes. Add the rest of the ingredients except the cilantro, put the lid on and cook on High for 15 minutes. Release the pressure naturally for 10 minutes, divide the mix between plates, sprinkle the cilantro on top and serve.

Nutrition: calories 231, fat 9.2, fiber 0.9, carbs 1.6, protein 33.6

Salsa Verde Turkey

Preparation time: 10 minutes | Cooking time: 30 minutes | Servings: 4

Ingredients:

- 1 big turkey breast, skinless, boneless and cubed
- 1 cup salsa Verde
- 1 cup chicken stock
- A pinch of salt and black pepper
- 1 tablespoon chives, chopped

Directions:

In your instant pot, combine all the ingredients, toss, put the lid on and cook on High for 30 minutes. Release the pressure naturally for 10 minutes, divide everything into bowls and serve,

Nutrition: calories 211, fat 6, fiber 0.3, carbs 2.8, protein 34.5

Basil Chicken Mix

Preparation time: 5 minutes | Cooking time: 25 minutes | Servings: 4

Ingredients:

- 2 chicken breasts, skinless, boneless and halved
- 1 cup chicken stock
- 1 and ½ tablespoons basil, chopped
- ¼ cup red bell peppers, cut into strips
- 4 garlic cloves, minced
- 1 tablespoon chili powder

Directions:

In your instant pot, combine the chicken with the rest of the ingredients, put the lid on and cook on High for 25 minutes. Release the pressure fast for 5 minutes, divide everything between plates and serve.

Nutrition: calories 230, fat 12.4, fiber 0.8, carbs 2.7, protein 33.2

Chicken and Hot Endives

Preparation time: 10 minutes | Cooking time: 25 minutes | Servings: 4

Ingredients:

- 2 chicken breasts, skinless, boneless and cubed
- 2 tablespoons ghee, melted
- 2 endives, shredded
- 1 teaspoon hot paprika
- 1 cup chicken stock
- 2 tablespoons tomato passata
- tablespoon dill, chopped

Directions:

Set the instant pot on Sauté mode, add the ghee, heat it up, add the meat and brown for 5 minutes. Add the other ingredients except the dill, put the lid on and cook on High for 20 minutes. Release the pressure naturally for 10 minutes, divide everything between plates and serve with the dill sprinkled on top.

Nutrition: calories 278, fat 15, fiber 0.2, carbs 1, protein 33.3

Indian Chicken and Sauce

Preparation time: 10 minutes | Cooking time: 30 minutes | Servings: 4

Ingredients:

- 2 chicken breasts, skinless, boneless and cubed
- 1 cup coconut cream
- A pinch of salt and black pepper
- 2 teaspoons garam masala
- 1 cup chicken stock
- ¼ cup cilantro, chopped

Directions:

In your instant pot, mix the chicken with rest of the ingredients, put the lid on and cook on High for 30 minutes. Release the pressure naturally for 10 minutes, divide everything between plates and serve.

Nutrition: calories 356, fat 22.9, fiber 1.4, carbs 3.6, protein 34.4

Turkey and Creamy Garlic Mix

Preparation time: 10 minutes | Cooking time: 25 minutes | Servings: 4

Ingredients:

- 1 big turkey breast, skinless, boneless and cubed
- 1 tablespoon ghee, melted
- 1 and ½ cups coconut cream
- A pinch of salt and black pepper
- 2 tablespoons tomato passata
- 2 tablespoons garlic, minced
- 1 teaspoon basil, dried

Directions:

Set your instant pot on Sauté mode, add the ghee, heat it up, add the meat and the garlic and brown for 5 minutes Add the rest of the ingredients, put the lid on and cook on High for 20 minutes. Release the pressure naturally for 10 minutes, divide between plates and serve.

Nutrition: calories 229, fat 8.9, fiber 0.2, carbs 1.8, protein 33.6

Chicken Casserole

Preparation time: 10 minutes | Cooking time: 30 minutes | Servings: 8

Ingredients:

- 2 pounds chicken breasts, skinless, boneless and cubed
- A pinch of salt and black pepper
- 2 tablespoons olive oil
- 2 scallions, chopped
- 1 pound Brussels sprouts, quartered
- 1 teaspoon sweet paprika
- 1 teaspoon thyme, dried
- ½ cup almonds, chopped

Directions:

Set your instant pot on Sauté mode, add the oil, heat it up, add the scallions and the meat and brown for 5 minutes. Add the remaining ingredients, put the lid on and cook on High for 25 minutes. Release the pressure naturally for 10 minutes, divide the casserole between plates and serve.

Nutrition: calories 307, fat 15.1, fiber 3.1, carbs 6.6, protein 36.1

Turkey and Cilantro Tomato Salsa

Preparation time: 10 minutes | Cooking time: 20 minutes | Servings: 4

Ingredients:

- 1 big turkey breast, skinless, boneless and cubed
- 1 cup tomatoes, cubed
- 1 tablespoon olive oil
- 1 avocado, peeled, pitted and cubed
- 2 spring onions, chopped
- 1 tablespoon cilantro, chopped
- A pinch of salt and black pepper
- 1 cup chicken stock
- 1 tablespoon smoked paprika

Directions:

Set your instant pot on Sauté mode, add the oil, heat it up, add the meat and brown for 5 minutes. Add the rest of the ingredients, put the lid on and cook on High for 20 minutes. Release the pressure naturally for 10 minutes, divide everything between plates and serve.

Nutrition: calories 343, fat 19.4, fiber 4.3, carbs 5.0, protein 34.5

Chicken and Green Sauté

Preparation time: 10 minutes | Cooking time: 30 minutes | Servings: 4

Ingredients:

- 1 shallot, chopped
- 1 pound chicken breast, skinless, boneless and sliced
- 1 cup kale, torn
- 1 cup mustard greens, torn
- 1 cup Brussels sprouts, shredded
- 1 cup chicken stock
- 2 tablespoons tomato passata
- 2 tablespoons olive oil
- 2 garlic cloves, minced
- A pinch of salt and black pepper

Directions:

Set your instant pot on Sauté mode, add the oil, heat it up, add the shallot and the meat and brown for 5 minutes Add the rest of the ingredients, put the lid on and cook on High for 25 minutes. Release the pressure naturally for 10 minutes, divide the mix between plates and serve.

Nutrition: calories 303, fat 15.7, fiber 1.7, carbs 5.6, protein 34.5

Chicken Meatballs and Spinach
Preparation time: 5 minutes | Cooking time: 30 minutes | Servings: 4

Ingredients:

- 1 pound chicken meat, ground
- 4 garlic cloves, minced
- 1 spring onion, chopped
- ¼ cup cilantro, chopped
- ½ cup coconut flour
- 1 egg, whisked
- A pinch of salt and black pepper
- 1 and ½ cups tomato passata
- tablespoons ghee, melted
- cups baby spinach
- 1 tablespoon parsley, chopped

Directions:

In a bowl, combine the meat with the garlic, onion, flour, cilantro, the egg, salt and pepper, stir well and shape medium meatballs out of this mix. Set the instant pot on Sauté mode, add the ghee, heat it up, add the meatballs and brown them for 2 minutes on each side. Add the sauce and the spinach, put the lid on and cook on High for 25 minutes. Release the pressure fast for 5 minutes, divide everything between plates and serve with the parsley sprinkled on top.

Nutrition: calories 297, fat 16, fiber 0.6, carbs 2, protein 35

Cheesy Turkey
Preparation time: 10 minutes | Cooking time: 25 minutes | Servings: 4

Ingredients:

- 1 turkey breast, skinless, boneless and cubed
- 1 tablespoon avocado oil
- 1 cup mozzarella, shredded
- cups mixed bell peppers, cut into strips
- 1 teaspoon chili powder
- 1 cup chicken stock
- 1 tablespoon cilantro, chopped

Directions:

Set the instant pot on Sauté mode, add the oil, heat it up, add the meat and chili powder and brown for 5 minutes. Add the rest of the ingredients except the cilantro and the mozzarella and toss gently. Sprinkle the mozzarella all over, put the lid on and cook on High for 20 minutes Release the pressure naturally for 10 minutes, divide everything between plates and serve with the cilantro sprinkled on top.

Nutrition: calories 222, fat 7.6, fiber 0.4, carbs 1, protein 35.5

Creamy Chicken Wings

Preparation time: 10 minutes | Cooking time: 30 minutes | Servings: 4

Ingredients:

- 1 pound chicken wings, halved
- 1 tablespoon olive oil
- tablespoons lemon juice
- garlic cloves, minced
- 1 cup chicken stock
- 1 cup heavy cream
- A pinch of salt and black pepper
- 1 tablespoon parsley, chopped

Directions:

Set your instant pot on Sauté mode, add the oil, heat it up, add the garlic and the chicken wings and brown for 5 minutes. Add the rest of the ingredients except the cream and the parsley, put the lid on and cook on High for 20 minutes. Release the pressure naturally for 10 minutes, set the pot on Sauté mode again, add the cream and parsley, toss, cook for 5 minutes, divide into bowls and serve.

Nutrition: calories 358, fat 23.2, fiber 0.1, carbs 2.3, protein 33.8

Turkey and Blackberries Sauce

Preparation time: 5 minutes | Cooking time: 30 minutes | Servings: 4

Ingredients:

- tablespoons olive oil
- 1 big turkey breast, skinless, boneless and cubed
- A pinch of salt and black pepper
- 1 cup blackberries
- 1 cup chicken stock
- shallots, minced
- 2 tablespoons chives, chopped

Directions:

Set your instant pot on sauté mode, add the oil, heat it up, add the meat and the shallots and brown for 5 minutes. Add the rest of the ingredients except the chives, put the lid on and cook on High for 25 minutes. Release the pressure fast for 5 minutes, divide everything between plates and serve with the chives sprinkled on top.

Nutrition: calories 271, fat 13, fiber 2, carbs 3.7, protein 33.9

Thyme Duck and Coconut
Preparation time: 10 minutes | Cooking time: 30 minutes | Servings: 6

Ingredients:

- 2 big duck legs, boneless, skinless and cubed
- 1 tablespoon olive oil
- 1 tablespoon thyme, chopped
- ½ cup coconut, unsweetened and shredded
- 1 cup coconut cream
- A pinch of salt and black pepper
- 1 cup chicken stock

Directions:

Set your instant pot on sauté mode, add the oil, heat it up, add the meat and brown for 5 minutes. Add the rest of the ingredients, put the lid on and cook on High for 25 minutes. Release the pressure naturally for 10 minutes, divide everything between plates and serve.

Nutrition: calories 273, fat 18.6, fiber 1.7, carbs 3.7, protein 23.3

Tuscan Chicken
Preparation time: 10 minutes | Cooking time: 25 minutes | Servings: 4

Ingredients:

- 1 pound chicken breast, skinless, boneless and cubed
- A pinch of salt and black pepper
- 1 tablespoon Italian seasoning
- 1 teaspoon oregano, dried
- tablespoons ghee, melted
- 1 cup cherry tomatoes, halved
- cups baby spinach
- 1 cup heavy cream
- ¼ cup parmesan, grated

Directions:

Set the instant pot on Sauté mode, add the ghee, heat it up, add the chicken and brown for 5 minutes. Add salt, pepper and the rest of the ingredients except the parmesan, put the lid on and cook on High for 20 minutes. Release the pressure naturally for 10 minutes, sprinkle the parmesan all over, divide between plates and serve.

Nutrition: calories 339, fat 22.4, fiber 1, carbs 3.8, protein 34.3

Marinated Turkey Mix

Preparation time: 5 minutes | Cooking time: 30 minutes | Servings: 6

Ingredients:

- 2 pounds turkey breast, skinless, boneless and cubed
- A pinch of salt and black pepper
- yellow bell peppers, cut into strips
- 2 shallots, chopped
- 1 broccoli head, florets separated
- ½ cup olive oil
- Juice of 2 limes
- ¼ cup cilantro, chopped

Directions:

Set your instant pot on Sauté mode, add the oil, heat it up, add the meat, lime juice and the cilantro and brown for 5 minutes. Add the rest of the ingredients, put the lid on and cook on High for 20 minutes. Release the pressure fast for 5 minutes, divide the mix between plates and serve.

Nutrition: calories 310, fat 18.4, fiber 0.4, carbs 2.3, protein 33.4

Tabasco Chicken and Kale

Preparation time: 10 minutes | Cooking time: 25 minutes | Servings: 4

Ingredients:

- 2 chicken breasts, skinless, boneless and cubed
- 2 tablespoons ghee, melted
- 1 tablespoon Tabasco sauce
- 2 cups kale, chopped
- A pinch of salt and black pepper
- 1 tablespoon basil, chopped
- 1 cup chicken stock

Directions:

Set your instant pot on sauté mode, add the ghee, heat it up, add the meat and brown for 5 minutes Add the rest of the ingredients, put the lid on and cook on High for 20 minutes. Release the pressure naturally for 10 minutes, divide everything between plates and serve.

Nutrition: calories 291, fat 14.9, fiber 0.5, carbs 3.8, protein 34.2

Chicken, Peppers and Mushrooms
Preparation time: 10 minutes | Cooking time: 25 minutes | Servings: 4

Ingredients:
- 2 chicken breasts, skinless, boneless and cubed
- 1 shallot, chopped
- 2 red bell peppers, cubed
- 2 green bell peppers, cubed
- 2 garlic cloves, minced
- 1 pound white mushrooms, halved
- A pinch of salt and black pepper
- 1 cup chicken stock

Directions:
In your instant pot, mix the chicken with the rest of the ingredients, put the lid on and cook on High for 25 minutes. Release the pressure naturally for 10 minutes, divide everything between plates and serve.

Nutrition: calories 283, fat 9.2, fiber 2.8, carbs 4.4, protein 34.5

Cheddar Turkey
Preparation time: 10 minutes | Cooking time: 30 minutes | Servings: 6

Ingredients:
- 1 tablespoon ginger, grated
- 4 garlic cloves, minced
- 1 tablespoon olive oil
- 1 cup coconut milk
- 1 big turkey breast, skinless, boneless and cubed
- A pinch of salt and black pepper
- 1 cup cheddar cheese, grated

Directions:
Set the instant pot on Sauté mode, add the oil, heat it up, add the garlic, ginger and the turkey and brown for 5 minutes. Add the rest of the ingredients except the cheese and toss. Sprinkle the cheese on top, put the lid on and cook on High for 25 minutes. Release the pressure naturally for 10 minutes, divide everything between plates and serve.

Nutrition: calories 323, fat 22, fiber 1, carbs 3.8, protein 28

Chicken and Almonds Mix

Preparation time: 5 minutes | Cooking time: 25 minutes | Servings: 4

Ingredients:

- 1 cup chicken stock
- 2 tablespoons avocado oil
- 2 chicken breasts, skinless, boneless and halved
- 1 tablespoon balsamic vinegar
- tablespoons almonds, chopped
- A pinch of salt and black pepper
- 1 tablespoon chives, chopped

Directions:

Set your instant pot on sauté mode, add the oil, heat it up, add the chicken and brown for 5 minutes. Add the rest of the ingredients, put the lid on and cook on High for 20 minutes. Release the pressure fast for 5 minutes, divide between plates and serve.

Nutrition: calories 254, fat 11.7, fiber 0.9, carbs 1.6, protein 34

Turkey, Brussels Sprouts and Walnuts

Preparation time: 5 minutes | Cooking time: 25 minutes | Servings: 4

Ingredients:

- 1 big turkey breast, skinless, boneless and cubed
- 1 tablespoon garlic, minced
- 2 tablespoons olive oil
- A pinch of salt and black pepper
- 1 tablespoon chili powder
- 1 pound Brussels sprouts, shredded
- 1 tablespoon walnuts, chopped

Directions:

Set your instant pot on sauté mode, add the oil, heat it up, add the meat and the garlic and brown for 5 minutes Add the rest of the ingredients, put the lid on and cook on High for 20 minutes. Release the pressure fast for 5 minutes, divide the mix between plates and serve.

Nutrition: calories 323, fat 14.5, fiber 5.4, carbs 6.3, protein 34.

Ketogenic Instant Pot Meat Recipes

Garlic and Parsley Pork
Preparation time: 10 minutes | Cooking time: 45 minutes | Servings: 6

Ingredients:

- 2 and ½ pounds pork shoulder, cubed
- 2 garlic cloves, minced
- 2 tablespoons parsley, chopped
- 1 teaspoon garlic powder
- 1 teaspoon oregano, dried
- 1 teaspoon rosemary, dried
- Salt and black pepper to the taste
- 2 cups beef stock

Directions:

In your instant pot, combine the pork with the garlic and the rest of the ingredients, put the lid on and cook on High for 45 minutes. Release the pressure naturally for 10 minutes, divide everything between plates and serve.

Nutrition: calories 454, fat 26.5, fiber 0.3, carbs 1.1, protein 35.6

Rosemary and Cinnamon Pork
Preparation time: 10 minutes | Cooking time: 40 minutes | Servings: 6

Ingredients:

- 1 and ½ pounds pork shoulder, cubed
- 1 tablespoon olive oil
- 1 cup beef stock
- 1 tablespoon rosemary, chopped
- 1 tablespoon cinnamon powder
- 2 garlic cloves, minced
- A pinch of salt and black pepper
- 1 teaspoon chili powder

Directions:

Set the instant pot on Sauté mode, add the oil, heat it up, add the meat, chili powder, rosemary and cinnamon and brown for 5 minutes. Add the remaining ingredients, toss, put the lid on and cook on High for 35 minutes. Release the pressure naturally for 10 minutes, divide the mix between plates and serve.

Nutrition: calories 352, fat 26.5, fiber 0.3, carbs 0.7, protein 26.5

Curry Pork and Kale

Preparation time: 10 minutes | Cooking time: 35 minutes | Servings: 6

Ingredients:

- 2 pounds pork shoulder, cubed
- 2 tablespoons avocado oil
- 2 tablespoons curry powder
- 1 pound kale, torn
- 2 garlic cloves, minced
- 1 cup beef stock
- 2 tablespoons parsley, chopped
- A pinch of salt and black pepper

Directions:

Set your instant pot on Sauté mode, add the oil, heat it up, add the meat, garlic and curry powder, toss and brown for 5 minutes. Add the rest of the ingredients, put the lid on and cook on High for 30 minutes. Release the pressure naturally for 10 minutes, divide everything between plates and serve.

Nutrition: calories 373, fat 25, fiber 1.6, carbs 6.9, protein 28.8

Pork and Cilantro Tomato Mix

Preparation time: 10 minutes | Cooking time: 35 minutes | Servings: 6

Ingredients:

- 1 and ½ pound pork stew meat, cubed
- 2 tablespoons olive oil
- 2 garlic cloves, minced
- 1 cup tomato passata
- 1 tablespoon cilantro, chopped
- ½ cup beef stock
- A pinch of salt and black pepper

Directions:

Set your instant pot on Sauté mode, add oil, heat it up, add the meat and the garlic and brown for 5 minutes. Add the rest of the ingredients, put the lid on and cook on High for 30 minutes. Release the pressure naturally for 10 minutes, divide the mix between plates and serve.

Nutrition: calories 285, fat 14.6, fiber 0.6, carbs 3.1, protein 33.9

Mustard Pork and Chard

Preparation time: 10 minutes | Cooking time: 40 minutes | Servings: 6

Ingredients:
- 1 and ½ pounds pork stew meat, cubed
- 1 tablespoon mustard
- 1 tablespoon ghee, melted
- 1 shallot, minced
- A pinch of salt and black pepper
- 1 pound red chard
- 2 garlic cloves, chopped
- 1 cup beef stock
- 1 tablespoon tomato passata
- 1 tablespoon parsley, chopped

Directions:
Set your instant pot on Sauté mode, add the ghee, heat it up, add the shallot, garlic, the meat and mustard, toss and brown for 5 minutes. Add the rest of the ingredients except the parsley, put the lid on and cook on High for 35 minutes. Release the pressure naturally for 10 minutes, divide the mix between plates, sprinkle the parsley on top and serve.

Nutrition: calories 353, fat 17.4, fiber 0.4, carbs 1.2, protein 34.2

Pork, Spinach and Green Beans

Preparation time: 10 minutes | Cooking time: 35 minutes | Servings: 6

Ingredients:
- 1 and ½ pound pork shoulder, cubed
- 1 shallot, minced
- ½ pound baby spinach
- 1 cup green beans, trimmed and halved
- 2 tablespoons olive oil
- A pinch of salt and black pepper
- ½ teaspoon chili powder
- 1 cup tomato passata
- 1 tablespoon parsley, chopped

Directions:
Set your instant pot on Sauté mode, add the oil, heat it up, add the meat, shallot and chili powder and brown for 5 minutes. Add the rest of the ingredients, put the lid on and cook on High for 30 minutes. Release the pressure naturally for 10 minutes, divide the mix between plates and serve.

Nutrition: calories 384, fat 26.5, fiber 1.8, carbs 5, protein 28.4

Pork, Kale and Capers Mix

Preparation time: 10 minutes | Cooking time: 40 minutes | Servings: 6

Ingredients:

- 2 pounds pork shoulder, cubed
- 1 tablespoon avocado oil
- 1 tablespoon capers, drained
- A pinch of salt and black pepper
- 1 cup beef stock
- 1 pound kale, torn
- ½ teaspoon smoked paprika
- 2 garlic cloves, minced
- 1 tablespoons chives, chopped
- 1 tablespoon oregano, chopped

Directions:

Set the instant pot on Sauté mode, add the oil, heat it up, add the meat, garlic and the paprika and brown for 5 minutes. Add the rest of the ingredients except the chives, put the lid on and cook on High for 35 minutes. Release the pressure naturally for 10 minutes, divide the mix between plates and serve with the chives sprinkled on top.

Nutrition: calories 367, fat 24.5, fiber 1.3, carbs 6.8, protein 28.2

Pork and Lemon Basil Sauce

Preparation time: 10 minutes | Cooking time: 30 minutes | Servings: 6

Ingredients:

- 2 tablespoons olive oil
- 1 and ½ pounds pork stew meat, cubed
- 2 tablespoons lemon juice
- 1 tablespoon lemon zest, grated
- 1 and ½ cup beef stock
- 2 tablespoons basil, chopped
- A pinch of salt and black pepper

Directions:

In your blender, combine the lemon zest with lemon juice, oil, stock and basil and pulse well. Set the instant pot on Sauté mode, add the basil sauce, heat it up, add the rest of the ingredients, toss, put the lid on and cook on High for 30 minutes. Release the pressure naturally for 10 minutes, divide the mix between plates and serve.

Nutrition: calories 272, fat 14.5, fiber 0.1, carbs 0.3, protein 33.3

Pork and Cauliflower Rice
Preparation time: 10 minutes | Cooking time: 30 minutes | Servings: 4

Ingredients:
- 1 pound pork shoulder, cubed
- 1 cup beef stock
- 1 cup cauliflower rice
- 2 tablespoons chives, chopped
- ½ teaspoon oregano, dried
- A pinch of salt and black pepper
- 2 tablespoons ghee, melted

Directions:
Set your instant pot on Sauté mode, add the ghee, heat it up, add the meat and brown for 5 minutes. Add the rest of the ingredients, put the lid on and cook on High for 25 minutes. Release the pressure naturally for 10 minutes, divide the mix between plates and serve.

Nutrition: calories 393, fat 13, fiber 0.1, carbs 0.2, protein 27.2

Spicy Pork, Zucchinis and Eggplants
Preparation time: 10 minutes | Cooking time: 30 minutes | Servings: 6

Ingredients:
- 1 and ½ pound pork shoulder, cubed
- 1 tablespoon olive oil
- 2 small zucchinis, sliced
- 2 small eggplants, cubed
- 1 tablespoon chili powder
- A pinch of red pepper flakes
- 2 spring onions, chopped
- 1 and ½ cups beef stock
- 1 tablespoon cilantro, chopped
- 2 tablespoons tomato paste
- A pinch of salt and black pepper

Directions:
Set your instant pot on Sauté mode, add the oil, heat it up, add the meat, chili powder and pepper flakes and brown for 5 minutes. Add the rest of the ingredients, put the lid on and cook on High for 25 minutes. Release the pressure naturally for 10 minutes, divide everything between plates and serve.

Nutrition: calories 396, fat 26.4, fiber 2.3, carbs 5.5, protein 28.5

Pork Meatballs and Spring Onions Sauce

Preparation time: 10 minutes | Cooking time: 25 minutes | Servings: 6

Ingredients:

- 2 tablespoons cilantro, chopped
- 1 and ½ pound pork, ground
- 1 cup beef stock
- 2 tablespoons tomato passata
- 1 egg, whisked
- 1 tablespoon olive oil
- ¼ teaspoon red pepper flakes
- A pinch of salt and black pepper
- 3 spring onions, chopped

Directions:

In a bowl, mix the pork with the cilantro, salt, pepper and the egg, stir well and shape medium meatballs out of this mix. Set the instant pot on Sauté mode, add the oil, heat it up, add the meatballs and brown for 2 minutes on each side. Add the rest of the ingredients, put the lid on and cook on High for 20 minutes. Release the pressure naturally for 10 minutes divide the mix between plates and serve.

Nutrition: calories 217, fat 7.4, fiber 0.3, carbs 0.8, protein 35.4

Raspberry Pork Mix

Preparation time: 10 minutes | Cooking time: 35 minutes | Servings: 4

Ingredients:

- 1 and ½ pounds pork shoulder, cubed
- 1 tablespoon ghee, melted
- 1 cup raspberries
- 1 cup beef stock
- 2 teaspoons sweet paprika
- 1 tablespoon chives, chopped
- 1 tablespoon balsamic vinegar

Directions:

Set your instant pot on Sauté mode, add the ghee, heat it up, add the meat and brown for 5 minutes. Add the rest of the ingredients, toss, put the lid on and cook on High for 20 minutes. Release the pressure naturally for 10 minutes, divide the mix between plates and serve.

Nutrition: calories 357, fat 23.3, fiber 1.2, carbs 2.2, protein 27.6

Chili Pork Chops

Preparation time: 10 minutes | Cooking time: 25 minutes | Servings: 4

Ingredients:

- 4 pork chops
- 1 tablespoon ghee, melted
- 1 cup beef stock
- 1 tablespoon chili powder
- 1 tablespoon sweet paprika
- 2 garlic cloves, chopped
- A pinch of salt and black pepper
- 1 tablespoon cilantro, chopped

Directions:

Set the instant pot on Sauté mode, add the ghee, heat it up, add the pork chops and brown for 2 minutes on each side. Add the rest of the ingredients, put the lid on and cook on High for 20 minutes. Release the pressure naturally for 10 minutes, divide the mix between plates and serve.

Nutrition: calories 303, fat 23.7, fiber 1.4, carbs 2.8, protein 19.4

Rosemary Pork Chops

Preparation time: 10 minutes | Cooking time: 30 minutes | Servings: 4

Ingredients:

- 4 pork chops
- 2 tablespoons avocado oil
- 2 garlic cloves, minced
- 2 tablespoons rosemary, chopped
- 1 and ½ cups beef stock
- A pinch of salt and black pepper
- 1 tablespoon chives, chopped

Directions:

Set your instant pot on Sauté mode, add the oil, heat it up, add the meat, garlic and rosemary and brown for 5 minutes. Add the rest of the ingredients, put the lid on and cook on High for 25 minutes. Release the pressure naturally for 10 minutes, divide everything between plates and serve.

Nutrition: calories 273, fat 21, fiber 1.1, carbs 2, protein 18.3

Pork Chops and Green Chilies Mix

Preparation time: 10 minutes | Cooking time: 25 minutes | Servings: 4

Ingredients:

- 4 pork chops
- 4 garlic cloves, minced
- 1 tablespoon cilantro, chopped
- 1 and ½ cups beef stock
- 2 tablespoons avocado oil
- 2 tablespoons tomato passata
- ½ cup canned green chilies, chopped
- A pinch of salt and black pepper

Directions:

Set your instant pot on Sauté mode, add the oil, heat it up, add the meat and the garlic and brown for 5 minutes. Add the rest of the ingredients, put the lid on and cook on High for 20 minutes. Release the pressure naturally for 10 minutes, divide the mix between plates and serve.

Nutrition: calories 287, fat 21.1, fiber 1.8, carbs 5.1, protein 18.9

Sage and Tarragon Pork

Preparation time: 10 minutes | Cooking time: 30 minutes | Servings: 4

Ingredients:

- 4 pork chops
- 2 tablespoons ghee, melted
- A pinch of salt and black pepper
- 1 teaspoon tarragon, dried
- 1 teaspoon sage, dried
- 2 garlic cloves, minced
- 2 cups beef stock
- 2 teaspoons sweet paprika

Directions:

Set your instant pot on Sauté mode, add the ghee, heat it up, add the meat and brown for 5 minutes. Add the rest of the ingredients, put the lid on and cook on High for 25 minutes. Release the pressure naturally for 10 minutes, divide the mix between plates and serve.

Nutrition: calories 328, fat 26.7, fiber 0.5, carbs 1.6, protein 19.7

Coconut Pork Mix

Preparation time: 10 minutes | Cooking time: 25 minutes | Servings: 6

Ingredients:

- 1 and ½ pounds pork shoulder, cubed
- ½ cup coconut cream
- 2 tablespoons sweet paprika
- 2 tablespoons ghee, melted
- 2 shallots, chopped
- A pinch of salt and black pepper
- 1 tablespoon parsley, chopped

Directions:

Set your instant pot on Sauté mode, add the ghee, heat it up, add the shallots and the meat and brown for 5 minutes. Add the rest of the ingredients, put the lid on and cook on High for 20 minutes. Release the pressure naturally for 10 minutes, divide the mix between plates and serve.

Nutrition: calories 321, fat 25.1, fiber 1, carbs 1.8, protein 21.7

Beef, Cauliflower Rice and Shrimp Mix

Preparation time: 10 minutes | Cooking time: 30 minutes | Servings: 4

Ingredients:

- 1 pound beef stew meat, cubed
- A pinch of salt and black pepper
- 2 tablespoons olive oil
- 1 cup cauliflower rice
- ½ pound shrimp, peeled and deveined
- 1 cup beef stock
- 12 ounces tomatoes, chopped
- 2 tablespoons cilantro, chopped

Directions:

Set your instant pot on Sauté mode, add the oil, heat it up, add the meat and brown for 5 minutes Add the rest of the ingredients except the shrimp, put the lid on and cook on High for 20 minutes. Release the pressure naturally for 10 minutes, set the pot on Sauté mode again, add the shrimp, cook for 5 minutes, divide the mix between plates and serve.

Nutrition: calories 358, fat 15.3, fiber 1, carbs 4.2, protein 38.2

Spiced Beef
Preparation time: 10 minutes | Cooking time: 30 minutes | Servings: 4

Ingredients:

- 2 pounds beef stew meat, cubed
- 1 tablespoon ghee, melted
- 1 cup veggie stock
- 2 spring onions, chopped
- 2 garlic cloves, minced
- A pinch of salt and black pepper
- 1 teaspoon allspice, ground
- 1 teaspoon turmeric powder
- 1 teaspoon ginger powder
- 1 teaspoon cinnamon powder

Directions:

Set the instant pot on Sauté mode, add the ghee, heat it up, add the meat, allspice, turmeric, ginger and the cinnamon and brown for 5 minutes. Add the rest of the ingredients, put the lid on and cook on High for 25 minutes. Release the pressure naturally for 10 minutes, divide the mix between plates and serve.

Nutrition: calories 306, fat 11.7, fiber 0.4, carbs 1.4, protein 45.4

Beef, Sprouts and Bok Choy Mix
Preparation time: 10 minutes | Cooking time: 30 minutes | Servings: 4

Ingredients:

- 1 and ½ pounds beef stew meat, cubed
- 1 cup bok choy, roughly chopped
- ¼ pound Brussels sprouts, shredded
- 1 cup tomato passata
- 2 garlic cloves, minced
- 2 tablespoons tomato paste
- 1 teaspoon olive oil
- A pinch of salt and black pepper
- 1 tablespoon chives, chopped

Directions:

Set your instant pot on Sauté mode, add the oil, heat it up, add the meat and the garlic and brown for 5 minutes. Add the rest of the ingredients except the chives, put the lid on and cook on High for 25 minutes. Release the pressure naturally for 10 minutes, divide everything between plates, sprinkle the chives on top and serve.

Nutrition: calories 319, fat 10.4, fiber 1.9, carbs 5.9, protein 26.5

Lamb and Broccoli Mix

Preparation time: 10 minutes | Cooking time: 25 minutes | Servings: 4

Ingredients:

- 1 and ½ cups broccoli florets
- 1 pound lamb shoulder, cubed
- 1 cup beef stock
- ¼ cup tomato passata
- 1 tablespoon dill chopped
- A pinch of salt and black pepper

Directions:

In your instant pot, mix the lamb with the stock and the rest of the ingredients, put the lid on and cook on High for 25 minutes. Release the pressure naturally for 10 minutes, divide the mix between plates and serve.

Nutrition: calories 234, fat 8.6, fiber 1.4, carbs 3.9, protein 34

Dill Lamb and Tomatoes

Preparation time: 10 minutes | Cooking time: 30 minutes | Servings: 4

Ingredients:

- 1 pound lamb shoulder, cubed
- 1 tablespoon olive oil
- 2 spring onions, chopped
- 2 cups tomato passata
- 2 garlic cloves, minced
- 1 tablespoon dill, chopped

Directions:

Set the instant pot on Sauté mode, add the oil, heat it up, add the lamb and brown for 5 minutes. Add the rest of the ingredients, put the lid on and cook on High for 25 minutes. Release the pressure naturally for 10 minutes, divide the mix between plates and serve.

Nutrition: calories 277, fat 12.1, fiber 2.2, carbs 5.9, protein 33.2

Curry Lamb and Cauliflower

Preparation time: 10 minutes | Cooking time: 40 minutes | Servings: 6

Ingredients:

- 2 pounds lamb shoulder, cubed
- 1 and ½ cups cauliflower florets
- 2 garlic cloves, minced
- 2 tablespoons ghee, melted
- 1 tablespoon curry powder
- 1 cup beef stock
- A pinch of salt and black pepper
- ½ bunch cilantro, chopped

Directions:

Set your instant pot on Sauté mode, add the ghee, heat it up, add the garlic and the lamb and brown for 5 minutes. Add the rest of the ingredients, put the lid on and cook on High for 35 minutes. Release the pressure naturally for 10 minutes, divide the mix between plates and serve.

Nutrition: calories 335, fat 15.6, fiber 1.2, carbs 2.7, protein 34.5

Garlic Lamb and Chard

Preparation time: 10 minutes | Cooking time: 35 minutes | Servings: 6

Ingredients:

- 2 pounds lamb shoulder, cubed
- 1 cup chard, chopped
- 3 garlic cloves, crushed
- A pinch of salt and black pepper
- 1 cup beef stock
- 2 tablespoons olive oil
- 1 tablespoon rosemary, chopped
- 1 tablespoon chives, chopped

Directions:

Set your instant pot on Sauté mode, add the oil, heat it up, add the garlic and the lamb and brown for 5 minutes. Add the rest of the ingredients except the chives, put the lid on and cook on High for 30 minutes. Release the pressure naturally for 10 minutes, divide the mix between plates and serve with the chives sprinkled on top.

Nutrition: calories 329, fat 16, fiber 0.4, carbs 1.1, protein 34.2

Coriander Beef and Pork Mix

Preparation time: 10 minutes | Cooking time: 35 minutes | Servings: 6

Ingredients:

- 1 pound beef stew meat, cubed
- 1 pound pork stew meat, cubed
- 2 tablespoons ghee, melted
- 1 tablespoon coriander, chopped
- A pinch of salt and black pepper
- 3 teaspoons turmeric powder
- 2 garlic cloves, minced
- 2 and ½ cups beef stock

Directions:

Set your instant pot on Sauté mode, add the ghee, heat it up, add the beef, the pork and the garlic and brown for 5 minutes Add the rest of the ingredients, put the lid on and cook on High for 30 minutes. Release the pressure naturally for 10 minutes, divide everything between plates and serve with a side salad.

Nutrition: calories 344, fat 16.4, fiber 0.3, carbs 1.1, protein 32.4

Pork Ribs and Green Beans

Preparation time: 10 minutes | Cooking time: 30 minutes | Servings: 4

Ingredients:

- 1 pound pork ribs rack
- ½ pound green beans, trimmed and halved
- 2 tablespoons olive oil
- 1 tablespoon smoked paprika
- 1 teaspoon chili powder
- A pinch of salt and black pepper
- 1 tablespoon rosemary, chopped
- ½ cup beef stock
- 1 tablespoon cilantro, chopped

Directions:

Set your instant pot on Sauté mode, add the oil, heat it up, add the meat, paprika and chili powder and brown for 5 minutes. Add the rest of the ingredients except the cilantro, put the lid on and cook on High for 25 minutes. Release the pressure naturally for 10, divide everything between plates and serve with the cilantro sprinkled on top.

Nutrition: calories 344, fat 21, fiber 3.2, carbs 5.9, protein 33.2

Lime Pork Chops

Preparation time: 5 minutes | Cooking time: 25 minutes | Servings: 4

Ingredients:

- 4 pork chops
- 2 tablespoons olive oil
- 2 garlic cloves, minced
- 2 tablespoons lime juice
- ½ cup tomato passata
- ½ cup beef stock
- A pinch of salt and black pepper
- 1 tablespoon cilantro, chopped

Directions:

Set your instant pot on Sauté mode, add the oil, heat it up, add the garlic and the pork chops and brown for 5 minutes. Add the rest of the ingredients except the cilantro, put the lid on and cook on High for 20 minutes. Release the pressure fast for 5 minutes, divide everything between plates and serve with the cilantro sprinkled on top.

Nutrition: calories 219, fat 18, fiber 0.3, carbs 1.5, protein 12.4

Pesto Pork and Mustard Greens

Preparation time: 10 minutes | Cooking time: 30 minutes | Servings: 4

Ingredients:

- 1 and ½ pounds pork shoulder, cubed
- 2 tablespoons ghee, melted
- ½ pound mustard greens, torn
- 1 cup beef stock
- 1 tablespoon basil pesto
- 2 garlic cloves, minced
- Salt and black pepper to the taste
- 1 tablespoon parsley, chopped

Directions:

Set the instant pot on Sauté mode, add the ghee, heat it up, add the meat and the garlic and brown for 5 minutes. Add the rest of the ingredients, toss, put the lid on and cook on High for 25 minutes. Release the pressure naturally for 10 minutes, divide the mix between plates and serve.

Nutrition: calories 370, fat 24.5, fiber 1, carbs 1.7, protein 27.5

Paprika Lamb Chops

Preparation time: 10 minutes | Cooking time: 30 minutes | Servings: 4

Ingredients:

- 4 lamb chops
- 1 tablespoon olive oil
- 1 cup tomatoes, cubed
- 1 cup beef stock
- 1 tablespoon sweet paprika
- A pinch of salt and black pepper
- 1 tablespoon rosemary, chopped

Directions:

Set the instant pot on Sauté mode, add the oil, heat it up, add the lamb and the paprika and brown for 5 minutes. Add the rest of the ingredients, toss, put the lid on and cook on High for 25 minutes. Release the pressure naturally for 10 minutes, divide everything between plates and serve.

Nutrition: calories 292, fat 13.2, fiber 1.6, carbs 3.3, protein 24.2

Pork and Olives

Preparation time: 10 minutes | Cooking time: 30 minutes | Servings: 6

Ingredients:

- 1 and ½ pounds pork shoulder, cubed
- 2 tablespoons ghee, melted
- A pinch of salt and black pepper
- 2 garlic cloves, minced
- 1 cup black olives, pitted and sliced
- 1 cup veggie stock
- ¼ cup tomato passata
- 1 tablespoon cilantro, chopped

Directions:

Set your instant pot on Sauté mode, add the ghee, heat it up, add the meat and the garlic and brown for 5 minutes. Add the rest of the ingredients except the cilantro, put the lid on and cook on High for 25 minutes. Release the pressure naturally for 10 minutes, divide the mix between plates and serve with the cilantro sprinkled on top.

Nutrition: calories 382, fat 23.2, fiber 0.7, carbs 1.7, protein 24.3

Beef and Herbed Radish

Preparation time: 10 minutes | Cooking time: 30 minutes | Servings: 4

Ingredients:

- 1 and ½ pound beef stew meat, cubed
- 1 cup radishes, sliced
- 1 tablespoon rosemary, chopped
- 1 tablespoon oregano, chopped
- 1 tablespoon basil, chopped
- 1 tablespoon olive oil
- 1 teaspoon sweet paprika
- 1 cup beef stock
- 1 tablespoon chives, chopped

Directions:

Set your instant pot on Sauté mode, add the oil, heat it up, add the meat and the paprika and brown for 5 minutes. Add the rest of the ingredients except the chives, put the lid on and cook on High for 50 minutes. Release the pressure naturally for 10 minutes, divide the mix between plates, sprinkle the chives on top and serve.

Nutrition: calories 312, fat 12.1, fiber 1, carbs 1.7, protein 24.2

Beef and Endives Mix

Preparation time: 10 minutes | Cooking time: 30 minutes | Servings: 4

Ingredients:

- 1 and ½ pounds beef stew meat, cubed
- 1 cup beef stock
- 2 endives, sliced
- 2 tablespoons lime juice
- 2 tablespoons ghee, melted
- 1 tablespoon cumin, ground
- 1 tablespoon sage, chopped
- 1 tablespoon sweet paprika
- A pinch of salt and black pepper

Directions:

Set the instant pot on Sauté mode, add the ghee, heat it up, add the meat and brown for 5 minutes. Add the rest of the ingredients, put the lid on and cook on High for 25 minutes. Release the pressure naturally for 10 minutes, divide the mix between plates and serve.

Nutrition: calories 329, fat 14.2, fiber 0.7, carbs 1.3, protein 23.4

Beef and Mushroom Rice

Preparation time: 10 minutes | Cooking time: 30 minutes | Servings: 4

Ingredients:

- 1 and ½ cups beef stock
- 1 tablespoon olive oil
- 1 and ½ pound beef stew meat, cubed
- 1 cup cauliflower rice
- 1 cup white mushrooms, halved
- 2 spring onions, chopped
- 2 teaspoons sweet paprika
- ¼ cup coconut cream
- 1 tablespoon chives, chopped
- A pinch of salt and black pepper

Directions:

Set your instant pot on sauté mode, add the oil, heat it up, add the spring onions, mushrooms and the beef and brown for 5 minutes Add the rest of the ingredients except the chives, put the lid on and cook on High for 25 minutes. Release the pressure naturally for 10 minutes, divide the mix between plates and serve with the chives sprinkled on top.

Nutrition: calories 336, fat 14.4, fiber 0.8, carbs 1.7, protein 23.2

Feta Cheese Lamb Mix

Preparation time: 10 minutes | Cooking time: 25 minutes | Servings: 4

Ingredients:

- 4 lamb chops
- 1 tablespoon olive oil
- ½ cup feta cheese, crumbled
- 1 cup kalamata olives, pitted and sliced
- 1 cup veggie stock
- 3 garlic cloves, minced
- 1 tablespoon rosemary, chopped
- 2 tablespoons tomato passata
- A pinch of salt and black pepper

Directions:

Set the instant pot on Sauté mode, add the oil, heat it up, add the lamb chops and brown for 2 minutes on each side. Add the rest of the ingredients except the cheese and the rosemary, put the lid on and cook on High for 20 minutes. Release the pressure naturally for 10 minutes, divide the mix between plates, sprinkle the cheese and the rosemary on top and serve.

Nutrition: calories 172, fat 13.2, fiber 1.6, carbs 4.6, protein 9.5

Mustard and Sage Beef

Preparation time: 10 minutes | Cooking time: 30 minutes | Servings: 4

Ingredients:

- 2 pounds beef stew meat, cubed
- A pinch of salt and black pepper
- 2 tablespoons Dijon mustard
- 1 tablespoon sage, chopped
- 1 tablespoon ghee, melted
- 1 cup tomato passata
- 1 cup beef stock
- 1 tablespoon parsley, chopped

Directions:

Set your instant pot on Sauté mode, add the ghee, heat it up, add the meat and brown for 5 minutes. Add the rest of the ingredients except the parsley, put the lid on and cook on High for 25 minutes. Release the pressure naturally for 10 minutes, divide mix between plates, sprinkle the parsley on top and serve.

Nutrition: calories 323, fat 12, fiber 1.1, carbs 4.3, protein 25.3

Spiced Lamb Meatballs

Preparation time: 10 minutes | Cooking time: 25 minutes | Servings: 4

Ingredients:

- 1 pound lamb shoulder, ground
- 1 tablespoon olive oil
- A pinch of salt and black pepper
- 1 teaspoon sweet paprika
- 1 and ½ cups tomato passata
- 1 teaspoon cinnamon powder
- 1 teaspoon cumin, ground
- 1 teaspoon coriander, ground
- 1 egg, whisked
- 1 tablespoon dill, chopped

Directions:

In a bowl, mix lamb meat with the rest of the ingredients except the tomato passata and the oil, stir well and shape medium meatballs put of this mix. Set the instant pot on Sauté mode, add the oil, heat it up, add the meatballs and cook them for 2 minutes on each side. Add the tomato passata, put the lid on and cook on High for 20 minutes. Release the pressure naturally for 10 minutes, divide meatballs and sauce between plates and serve.

Nutrition: calories 262, fat 13.1, fiber 0.4, carbs 1.1, protein 33.2

Mint Lamb Chops

Preparation time: 10 minutes | Cooking time: 25 minutes | Servings: 4

Ingredients:

- ½ cup cilantro, chopped
- 4 lamb chops
- 2 green chilies, chopped
- 3 garlic cloves, minced
- Juice of 2 limes
- 2 tablespoons olive oil
- A pinch of salt and black pepper
- ½ cup mint, chopped
- 1 cup veggie stock

Directions:

Set your instant pot on Sauté mode, add the oil, heat it up, add the garlic, chilies and the lamb chops and brown for 5 minutes Add the rest of the ingredients, put the lid on and cook on High for 25 minutes. Release the pressure naturally for 10 minutes, divide the mix between plates and serve.

Nutrition: calories 143, fat 10.9, fiber 0.9, carbs 3, protein 15.6

Lamb Chops, Fennel and Tomatoes

Preparation time: 10 minutes | Cooking time: 25 minutes | Servings: 4

Ingredients:

- 4 lamb chops
- 1 tablespoon olive oil
- 4 garlic cloves, minced
- A pinch of salt and black pepper
- Zest of 1 lime, grated
- 2 bay leaves
- 1 tablespoon rosemary, chopped
- 1 fennel bulb, cut into 8 wedges
- ½ cup cherry tomatoes, halved
- 1 teaspoon sweet paprika
- 1 cup veggie stock

Directions:

Set your instant pot on Sauté mode, add the oil, heat it up, add the meat and the garlic and brown for 5 minutes. Add the rest of the ingredients, put the lid on and cook on High for 20 minutes. Release the pressure naturally for 10 minutes, divide everything between plates and serve.

Nutrition: calories 194, fat 7.9, fiber 2.3, carbs 5.3, protein 7.5

Italian Leg of Lamb

Preparation time: 10 minutes | Cooking time: 40 minutes | Servings: 4

Ingredients:

- 2 pounds leg of lamb, boneless
- 2 tablespoons olive oil
- 4 garlic cloves, minced
- 2 tablespoons rosemary, chopped
- ¼ teaspoon red pepper flakes
- ½ cup walnuts, chopped
- 5 ounces baby spinach
- A pinch of salt and black pepper
- ½ cup mustard

Directions:

Set your instant pot on Sauté mode, add the oil, heat it up, add the garlic, pepper flakes, the lamb and the mustard, toss and cook for 5 minutes. Add all the other ingredients except the spinach, put the lid on and cook on High for 30 minutes. Release the pressure naturally for 10 minutes, set the pot on Sauté mode again, add the spinach, cook for 5 minutes more, divide the mix between plates and serve.

Nutrition: calories 367, fat 25.3, fiber 3.5, carbs 5.8, protein 25.4

Hot Curry Lamb and Green Beans

Preparation time: 10 minutes | Cooking time: 35 minutes | Servings: 4

Ingredients:

- 4 lamb chops
- 1 pound green beans, trimmed and halved
- Juice of 1 lime
- A pinch of salt and black pepper
- ½ cup beef stock
- 1 teaspoon rosemary, dried
- 1 tablespoon olive oil
- 1 tablespoon curry powder

Directions:

In your instant pot, combine all the ingredients, put the lid on and cook on High for 35 minutes. Release the pressure naturally for 10 minutes, divide the mix between plates and serve.

Nutrition: calories 139, fat 7.7, fiber 3.4, carbs 4.6, protein 8.9

Lamb and Sun-dried Tomatoes Mix

Preparation time: 10 minutes | Cooking time: 40 minutes | Servings: 6

Ingredients:

- 6 lamb loins
- 2 garlic cloves, minced
- 2 teaspoons thyme, chopped
- A pinch of salt and black pepper
- 2 tablespoons olive oil
- 2 tablespoons balsamic vinegar
- ½ cup parsley, chopped
- ½ cup sun-dried tomatoes, chopped
- 1 cup beef stock

Directions:

Set the instant pot on Sauté mode, add the oil, heat it up, add the lamb and garlic and brown for 5 minutes. Add the rest of the ingredients, put the lid on and cook on High for 35 minutes. Release the pressure naturally for 10 minutes, divide the mix between plates and serve.

Nutrition: calories 353, fat 23.7, fiber 0.5, carbs 1.5, protein 34.2

Cumin Lamb and Capers

Preparation time: 10 minutes | Cooking time: 35 minutes | Servings: 4

Ingredients:

- 4 lamb chops
- 2 tablespoons avocado oil
- A pinch of salt and black pepper
- 2 tablespoons sweet paprika
- 2 tablespoons capers, drained
- 1 cup beef stock
- 2 teaspoons cumin, ground
- 1 tablespoon parsley, chopped
- 1 tablespoon cilantro, chopped

Directions:

Set the instant pot on Sauté mode, add the oil, heat it up, add the lamb chops, paprika and cumin and brown for 5 minutes. Add the rest of the ingredients, put the lid on and cook on High for 30 minutes. Release the pressure naturally for 10 minutes, divide the mix between plates and serve.

Nutrition: calories 110, fat 5.6, fiber 1.9, carbs 4.5, protein 7.9

Herbed Crusted Lamb Cutlets

Preparation time: 10 minutes | Cooking time: 30 minutes | Servings: 4

Ingredients:

- 8 lamb cutlets
- 4 tablespoons mustard
- 3 tablespoons olive oil
- ¼ cup parmesan, grated
- 1 tablespoon parsley, chopped
- 1 tablespoon thyme, chopped
- 1 tablespoon rosemary
- 1 cup tomato passata

Directions:

In a bowl, mix the lamb with the rest of the ingredients except the tomato passata. Add the sauce to the instant pot, add the lamb, put the lid on and cook on High for 30 minutes. Release the pressure naturally for 10 minutes, divide the mix between plates and serve.

Nutrition: calories 162, fat 14, fiber 3.3, carbs 6.5, protein 14.4

Pine Nuts Lamb Meatballs

Preparation time: 10 minutes | Cooking time: 30 minutes | Servings: 6

Ingredients:

- 2 pounds lamb, ground
- ½ cup almond milk
- 2 shallots, minced
- 2 garlic cloves, minced
- 1 tablespoon thyme, chopped
- A pinch of salt and black pepper
- ½ cup pine nuts, toasted
- 1 egg
- 1 tablespoon olive oil
- 12 ounces canned tomatoes, crushed

Directions:

In a bowl, combine the lamb with the rest of the ingredients except the oil and the tomatoes, stir well and shape medium meatballs out of this mix Set the instant pot on Sauté mode, add the oil, heat it up, add the meatballs and cook for 2 minutes on each side. Add the tomatoes, put the lid on and cook on High for 25 minutes. Release the pressure naturally for 10 minutes, divide the mix between plates and serve.

Nutrition: calories 363, fat 26.4, fiber 1.6, carbs 5.5, protein 24.8

Lamb Shoulder Roast

Preparation time: 10 minutes | Cooking time: 35 minutes | Servings: 6

Ingredients:

- 2 tablespoons ghee, melted
- 2 tablespoons olive oil
- 2 shallots, chopped
- 2 garlic cloves, minced
- ½ cup mint, chopped
- 2 pounds lamb shoulder, fat trimmed
- 1 cup veggie stock

Directions:

Set the instant pot on Sauté mode, add the oil and the ghee, heat it up, add the lamb shoulder, garlic and shallots and sear for 2 minutes on each side. Add all the other ingredients, put the lid on and cook on High for 30 minutes. Release the pressure naturally for 10 minutes, slice the roast, between plates and serve.

Nutrition: calories 378, fat 19.2, fiber 0.4, carbs 0.7, protein 27.5

Moroccan Lamb

Preparation time: 10 minutes | Cooking time: 30 minutes | Servings: 4

Ingredients:
- 8 lamb chops
- 1 cup Greek yogurt
- 3 tablespoons olive oil
- 1 tablespoon lemon zest, grated
- A pinch of salt and black pepper
- 1 tablespoon cumin, ground
- 1 tablespoon coriander, ground
- 1 tablespoon turmeric powder
- ½ cup mint, chopped
- 4 garlic cloves, minced
- 2 tablespoons lemon juice
- 1 and ½ cups veggie stock

Directions:

Set the instant pot on Sauté mode, add the oil, heat it up, add the meat, cumin, coriander and turmeric and brown for 5 minutes. Add the rest of the ingredients, put the lid on and cook on High for 25 minutes. Release the pressure naturally for 10 minutes, divide everything between plates and serve.

Nutrition: calories 179, fat 14.9, fiber 1.5, carbs 5.5, protein 7.5

Spinach Pork Meatloaf

Preparation time: 10 minutes | Cooking time: 30 minutes | Servings: 6

Ingredients:
- ½ cup almond milk
- ½ cup almond flour
- 1 spring onion, chopped
- A pinch of salt and black pepper
- 2 eggs, whisked
- 1 cup baby spinach
- 2 pounds pork meat, ground
- ½ cup tomato passata
- 1 tablespoon parsley, chopped
- 1 and ½ cups water

Directions:

In a bowl, mix pork with the rest of the ingredients except the tomato passata and the water, stir well, transfer to a loaf pan that fits the instant pot and brush it with the tomato passata. Add the water to your instant pot, add the steamer basket, put the loaf pan inside, put the lid on and cook on High for 30 minutes. Release the pressure naturally for 10 minutes, cool the meatloaf down, slice and serve.

Nutrition: calories 394, fat 26.8, fiber 1, carbs 2.7, protein 35.6

Ginger Lamb and Basil

Preparation time: 10 minutes | Cooking time: 30 minutes | Servings: 4

Ingredients:

- 1 and ½ pounds leg of lamb, boneless and cubed
- 1 tablespoon olive oil
- 2 tablespoons basil, chopped
- 1 tablespoon ginger, grated
- A pinch of salt and black pepper
- 1 and ½ cups veggie stock
- 1 cup tomato passata

Directions:

Set the instant pot on Sauté mode, add the oil, heat it up, add the meat and brown for 5 minutes. Add the rest of the ingredients, put the lid on and cook on High for 25 minutes. Release the pressure naturally for 10 minutes, divide the mix between plates and serve.

Nutrition: calories 320, fat 13.6, fiber 0.9, carbs 4.4, protein 35.6

Coconut Lamb Chops

Preparation time: 10 minutes | Cooking time: 30 minutes | Servings: 6

Ingredients:

- 6 lamb chops
- 2 tablespoons olive oil
- 1 teaspoon rosemary, chopped
- 1 cup veggie stock
- 1 tablespoon garlic, minced
- A pinch of salt and black pepper
- 1 cup coconut cream
- 1 tablespoon dill, chopped

Directions:

Set the instant pot on Sauté mode, add the oil, heat it up, add the lamb, garlic and rosemary and brown for 5 minutes. Add the rest of the ingredients, put the lid on and cook on High for 25 minutes. Release the pressure naturally for 10 minutes, divide everything between plates and serve.

Nutrition: calories 269, fat 25.1, fiber 1.6, carbs 5.9, protein 7.9

Spicy Beef, Sprouts and Avocado Mix

Preparation time: 10 minutes | Cooking time: 30 minutes | Servings: 4

Ingredients:

- 1 pound beef stew meat, cubed
- 1 avocado, peeled, pitted and cubed
- 2 cups Brussels sprouts, trimmed and quartered
- ½ teaspoon oregano, dried
- A pinch of salt and black pepper
- 1 tablespoon avocado oil
- 1 cup beef stock
- 1 teaspoon sweet paprika

Directions:

Set the instant pot on Sauté mode, add the oil, heat it up, add the meat, oregano, paprika, salt and pepper and brown for 5 minutes Add the rest of the ingredients except the avocado, put the lid on and cook on High for 25 minutes. Release the pressure naturally for 10 minutes, divide the mix between plates and serve with the avocado on top.

Nutrition: calories 343, fat 17.5, fiber 3.3, carbs 6.7, protein 34.8

Beef and Creamy Sauce

Preparation time: 10 minutes | Cooking time: 35 minutes | Servings: 6

Ingredients:

- 2 pounds beef stew meat, cubed
- 2 shallots, minced
- 1 cup coconut cream
- ½ teaspoon rosemary, chopped
- 1 tablespoon olive oil
- 1 cup beef stock
- 1 tablespoon dill, chopped
- A pinch of salt and black pepper

Directions:

Set your instant pot on Sauté mode, add the oil, heat it up, add the meat, shallots and the rosemary and brown for 5 minutes. Add rest of the ingredients except the cream, put the lid on and cook on High for 25 minutes. Release the pressure naturally for 10 minutes, set the pot on Sauté mode again, add the cream, toss and cook for 10 minutes more. Divide the mix between plates and serve.

Nutrition: calories 397, fat 21.4, fiber 1, carbs 2.6, protein 32.4

Pork and Chives Asparagus

Preparation time: 10 minutes | Cooking time: 30 minutes | Servings: 6

Ingredients:

- 2 pounds pork stew meat, cubed
- 4 garlic cloves, minced
- 1 cup beef stock
- 1 bunch asparagus, trimmed
- A pinch of salt and black pepper
- 1 teaspoon sweet paprika
- 1 teaspoon chives, chopped
- 1 tablespoon olive oil

Directions:

Set your instant pot on sauté mode, add the oil, heat it up, add the garlic and the beef stew meat and brown for 5 minutes Add the rest of the ingredients except the asparagus, put the lid on and cook on High for 20 minutes. Release the pressure naturally for 10 minutes, set the pot on Sauté mode again, add the asparagus, cook for 5 minutes more, divide everything between plates and serve.

Nutrition: calories 347, fat 17.1, fiber 0.2, carbs 0.9, protein 24.7

Oregano and Thyme Beef

Preparation time: 5 minutes | Cooking time: 30 minutes | Servings: 4

Ingredients:

- 1 pound beef stew meat, cubed
- 2 garlic cloves, minced
- 1 tablespoon olive oil
- 1 teaspoon thyme, dried
- A pinch of salt and black pepper
- 1 tablespoon oregano, chopped
- 1 and ½ cups beef stock

Directions:

Set your instant pot on Sauté mode, add the oil, heat it up, add the garlic, thyme and the meat and brown for 5 minutes. Add the rest of the ingredients, put the lid on and cook on High for 25 minutes. Release the pressure naturally for 10 minutes, divide the mix between plates and serve.

Nutrition: calories 247, fat 10.7, fiber 0.6, carbs 1.4, protein 34.2

Almond Lamb Meatloaf

Preparation time: 10 minutes | Cooking time: 30 minutes | Servings: 4

Ingredients:

- 1 and ½ pound lamb, ground
- 2 shallots, minced
- 2 eggs, whisked
- 3 garlic cloves, minced
- 1 tablespoon almonds, chopped
- 1 tablespoon rosemary
- A pinch of salt and black pepper
- 1 cup kale, chopped
- ¼ cup coconut milk
- Cooking spray
- 2 cups water

Directions:

In a bowl, combine the meat with rest of the ingredients except the cooking spray and the water, and stir well. Grease a loaf pan that fits the instant pot with the cooking spray, shape the meatloaf and put it in the pan. Add the water to the instant pot, add the steamer basket, put the meatloaf inside, put the lid on and cook on High for 30 minutes. Release the pressure naturally for 10 minutes, cool the meatloaf, slice and serve.

Nutrition: calories 301, fat 15.1, fiber 1.2, carbs 4.4, protein 35.4

Pork and Bok Choy

Preparation time: 10 minutes | Cooking time: 35 minutes | Servings: 6

Ingredients:

- 1 and ½ pounds pork stew meat, cubed
- 4 garlic cloves, minced
- 2 tablespoons chili powder
- 1 teaspoon red pepper flakes
- 1 pound bok choy, torn
- 1 tablespoon olive oil
- A pinch of salt and black pepper
- 1 cup beef stock

Directions:

Set the instant pot on sauté mode, add the oil, heat it up, add the garlic, the meat, chili powder and pepper flakes and brown for 5 minutes. Add the rest of the ingredients, put the lid on and cook on High for 30 minutes. Release the pressure naturally for 10 minutes, divide the mix between plates and serve.

Nutrition: calories 365, fat 17.5, fiber 1.8, carbs 3.9, protein 34.6

Smoked Paprika Lamb

Preparation time: 10 minutes | Cooking time: 30 minutes | Servings: 4

Ingredients:

- 1 and ½ pounds leg of lamb, boneless and cubed
- 1 tablespoon smoked paprika
- 1 and ½ cups tomatoes, cubed
- 3 garlic cloves, minced
- 1 cup veggie stock
- 1 tablespoon ghee, melted
- A pinch of salt and black pepper
- 1 tablespoon cilantro, chopped

Directions:

Set your instant pot on Sauté mode, add the ghee, heat it up, add the meat, smoked paprika and the garlic and brown for 6 minutes. Add the rest of the ingredients except the cilantro, put the lid on and cook on High for 25 minutes. Release the pressure naturally for 10 minutes, divide the mix between plates and serve with the cilantro sprinkled on top.

Nutrition: calories 306, fat 13.4, fiber 0.5, carbs 1.2, protein 43.2

Cajun Beef and Leeks Sauce

Preparation time: 10 minutes | Cooking time: 35 minutes | Servings: 6

Ingredients:

- 2 pounds beef sirloin, cut into steaks
- 1 tablespoon olive oil
- 2 tablespoons Cajun seasoning
- 1 and ½ cups beef stock
- A pinch of salt and black pepper
- 1 teaspoon garlic, minced
- 1 leek, sliced

Directions:

Set your instant pot on sauté mode, add the oil, heat it up, add the garlic, the meat and Cajun seasoning and brown for 5 minutes. Add the remaining ingredients, put the lid on and cook on High for 30 minutes. Release the pressure naturally for 10 minutes, divide the mix between plates and serve.

Nutrition: calories 311, fat 11.8, fiber 0.3, carbs 2.3, protein 25.7

Beef and Savoy Cabbage Mix

Preparation time: 10 minutes | Cooking time: 25 minutes | Servings: 4

Ingredients:

- 1 pound beef stew meat, cubed
- 1 Savoy cabbage, shredded
- 2 garlic cloves, minced
- 1 tablespoon olive oil
- A pinch of salt and black pepper
- 1 and ½ cups tomato passata
- 1 tablespoon parsley, chopped

Directions:

Set the instant pot on Sauté mode, add the oil, heat it up, add the meat and the garlic and brown for 5 minutes. Add the rest of the ingredients, put the lid on and cook on High for 20 minutes. Release the pressure naturally for 10 minutes, divide the mix between plates and serve.

Nutrition: calories 243, fat 10.6, fiber 0.1, carbs 0.6, protein 34.5

Pork and Mint Zucchinis

Preparation time: 10 minutes | Cooking time: 25 minutes | Servings: 6

Ingredients:

- 2 pounds pork stew meat, cubed
- A pinch of salt and black pepper
- 1 cup beef stock
- 1 cup zucchinis, sliced
- 1 tablespoon balsamic vinegar
- 1 tablespoon olive oil
- 1 tablespoon garlic, minced
- 1 tablespoon mint, chopped

Directions:

Set the instant pot on Sauté mode, add the oil, heat it up, add the pork and the garlic and brown for 5 minutes. Add the rest of the ingredients, put the lid on and cook on High for 20 minutes. Release the pressure naturally for 10 minutes, divide everything between plates and serve.

Nutrition: calories 349, fat 17.1, fiber 0.3, carbs 1.2, protein 34.2

Beef and Walnuts Rice

Preparation time: 10 minutes | Cooking time: 35 minutes | Servings: 6

Ingredients:

- 1 and ½ pounds beef stew meat, cubed
- 2 garlic cloves, minced
- 1 cup beef stock
- 1 tablespoon walnuts, toasted and chopped
- 1 cup tomato passata
- A pinch of salt and black pepper
- 1 tablespoon basil, chopped
- 1 tablespoon olive oil

Directions:

Set your instant pot on sauté mode, add the oil, heat it up, add the meat and the garlic and brown for 5 minutes. Add the rest of the ingredients, put the lid on and cook on High for 30 minutes. Release the pressure naturally for 10 minutes, divide everything between plates and serve.

Nutrition: calories 329, fat 12.7, fiber 0.9, carbs 4.2, protein 27.6

Ketogenic Instant Pot Vegetable Recipes

Lime and Paprika Asparagus

Preparation time: 5 minutes | Cooking time: 15 minutes | Servings: 4

Ingredients:

- 2 pounds asparagus, trimmed
- 1 tablespoon lime juice
- 1 tablespoon lime zest, grated
- 1 tablespoon sweet paprika
- 2 cups chicken stock
- A pinch of salt and black pepper

Directions:

In your instant pot, combine the asparagus with the rest of the ingredients, put the lid on and cook on High for 15 minutes. Release the pressure fast for 5 minutes, divide between plates and serve.

Nutrition: calories 56, fat 1.8, fiber 0.4, carbs 0.5, protein 5.6

Basil Spicy Artichokes

Preparation time: 10 minutes | Cooking time: 20 minutes | Servings: 4

Ingredients:

- 4 big artichokes, trimmed
- A pinch of salt and black pepper
- ¼ cup chicken stock
- 1 teaspoon basil, chopped
- ½ teaspoon hot paprika
- A pinch of red pepper flakes
- A pinch of cayenne pepper

Directions:

In your instant pot, combine the artichokes with the rest of the ingredients, put the lid on and cook on High for 20 minutes. Release the pressure naturally for 10 minutes, divide the artichokes between plates and serve.

Nutrition: calories 10, fat 1.1, fiber 0.8, carbs 1.6, protein 0.6

Coconut Leeks and Sprouts

Preparation time: 5 minutes | Cooking time: 20 minutes | Servings: 4

Ingredients:

- 2 leeks, sliced
- 1 pound Brussels sprouts, halved
- ½ cup chicken stock
- ½ cup coconut cream
- 1 tablespoon dill, chopped
- A pinch of salt and black pepper

Directions:

In your instant pot, combine leeks with the sprouts and the rest of the ingredients, put the lid on and cook on High for 20 minutes. Release the pressure fast for 5 minutes, divide the mix between plates and serve.

Nutrition: calories 148, fat 7.8, fiber 2.9, carbs 5.4, protein 5.5

Mozzarella Artichokes and Capers
Preparation time: 5 minutes | Cooking time: 15 minutes | Servings: 4

Ingredients:
- 4 artichokes, trimmed
- 1 cup chicken stock
- 1 tablespoon sweet paprika
- 1 tablespoon capers, drained
- 1 tablespoon basil, chopped
- 2 garlic cloves, chopped
- 1 cup mozzarella, shredded

Directions:
In your instant pot, combine the artichokes with the rest of the ingredients except the mozzarella, put the lid on and cook on High for 15 minutes. Release the pressure fast for 5 minutes, divide the mix between plates, sprinkle the mozzarella on top and serve.

Nutrition: calories 106, fat 1.9, fiber 0.2, carbs 0.5, protein 7.8

Asparagus and Tomatoes
Preparation time: 5 minutes | Cooking time: 15 minutes | Servings: 4

Ingredients:
- 1 pound asparagus, trimmed
- 1 cup chicken stock
- A pinch of salt and black pepper
- 2 cups cherry tomatoes, halved
- 1 tablespoon basil, chopped
- 1 tablespoon chives, chopped

Directions:
In your instant pot, mix the asparagus with the stock and the rest of the ingredients, put the lid on and cook on High for 15 minutes. Release the pressure fast for 5 minutes, divide mix between plates and serve.

Nutrition: calories 42, fat 1.2, fiber 0.7, carbs 1, protein 3.5

Asparagus and Chives Dressing

Preparation time: 5 minutes | Cooking time: 10 minutes | Servings: 4

Ingredients:

- 1 pound asparagus, trimmed
- 2 tablespoons olive oil
- 2 cups water
- A pinch of salt and black pepper
- 1 teaspoon garlic powder
- 1 cup avocado mayonnaise
- 1 cup Greek yogurt
- 1 and ½ cups basil, chopped
- ½ cup parsley, chopped
- ¼ cup chives, chopped
- ¼ cup lemon juice

Directions:

Put the water in the instant pot, add the steamer basket, add the asparagus inside, put the lid on and cook on High for 10 minutes. Release the pressure fast for 5 minutes, and divide the asparagus between plates. In a blender, mix the avocado mayonnaise with the rest of the ingredients, pulse well, spread over the asparagus and serve.

Nutrition: calories 102, fat 7.5, fiber 3, carbs 6.1, protein 3.4

Creamy Asparagus Mix

Preparation time: 5 minutes | Cooking time: 10 minutes | Servings: 4

Ingredients:

- 1 bunch asparagus, trimmed
- 2 tablespoons oregano, chopped
- 1 cup heavy cream
- A pinch of salt and black pepper
- 1 cup chicken stock

Directions:

In your instant pot, mix the asparagus with the rest of the ingredients, put the lid on and cook on High for 10 minutes. Release the pressure fast for 5 minutes, divide everything between plates and serve.

Nutrition: calories 121, fat 11.5, fiber 1.8, carbs 4.1, protein 1.9

Parmesan Radishes and Asparagus

Preparation time: 5 minutes | Cooking time: 10 minutes | Servings: 4

Ingredients:

- 1 bunch asparagus, trimmed
- 2 cups radishes, sliced
- 1 cup chicken stock
- 1 tablespoon chives, chopped
- 1 teaspoon chili powder

Directions:

In your instant pot, combine the asparagus with the radishes and the rest of the ingredients, put the lid on and cook on High for 10 minutes. Release the pressure fast for 5 minutes, divide the mix between plates and serve.

Nutrition: calories 45, fat 0.6, fiber 0.1, carbs 0.4, protein 2

Artichokes and Bacon Mix

Preparation time: 5 minutes | Cooking time: 10 minutes | Servings: 4

Ingredients:

- 4 artichokes, trimmed
- 2 teaspoons lemon zest, grated
- 1 cup chicken stock
- 1 cup bacon, cooked and crumbled
- 1 teaspoon chili powder
- A pinch of salt and black pepper
- 1 tablespoon basil, chopped
- 1 tablespoon parsley, chopped

Directions:

In your instant pot, combine the artichokes with the lemon zest and the rest of the ingredients except the bacon, put the lid on and cook on High for 10 minutes. Release the pressure fast for 5 minutes, divide the mix between plates, sprinkle the bacon on top and serve.

Nutrition: calories 82, fat 2.5, fiber 1.9, carbs 2.1, protein 5.6

Balsamic Green Beans and Capers

Preparation time: 10 minutes | Cooking time: 20 minutes | Servings: 4

Ingredients:

- 1 and ½ cups chicken stock
- 1 pound green beans, trimmed and halved
- 1 tablespoon capers, drained
- A pinch of salt and black pepper
- 2 garlic cloves, minced
- 1 tablespoon dill, chopped
- 1 tablespoon balsamic vinegar

Directions:

In your instant pot, combine the green beans with the stock and the rest of the ingredients, put the lid on and cook on High for 20 minutes. Release the pressure naturally for 10 minutes, divide everything between plates and serve.

Nutrition: calories 46, fat 1.7, fiber 0.1, carbs 0.6, protein 2.7

Brussels Sprouts and Sauce

Preparation time: 5 minutes | Cooking time: 20 minutes | Servings: 4

Ingredients:

- 1 pound Brussels sprouts, trimmed and halved
- 1 cup chicken stock
- 2 garlic cloves, minced
- A pinch of salt and black pepper
- 1 tablespoon dill, chopped
- 1 tablespoon heavy cream
- 1 tablespoon rosemary, chopped

Directions:

In your instant pot, mix the sprouts with the stock and the rest of the ingredients, put the lid on and cook on High for 20 minutes. Release the pressure fast for 5 minutes, divide the mix between plates and serve.

Nutrition: calories 71, fat 2.1, fiber 1.1, carbs 1.3, protein 4.4

Bell Peppers and Chives

Preparation time: 10 minutes | Cooking time: 20 minutes | Servings: 4

Ingredients:

- 1 pound red bell peppers, cut into wedges
- 1 cup veggie stock
- 1 tablespoon chives, chopped
- 1 tablespoon sweet paprika
- 1 tablespoon chives, chopped

Directions:

In your instant pot, mix the bell peppers with the rest of the ingredients except the chives, put the lid on and cook on High for 20 minutes. Release the pressure naturally for 10 minutes, divide the mix between plates and serve with the chives sprinkled on top.

Nutrition: calories 70, fat 1.8, fiber 1.1, carbs 1.4, protein 0.6

Cayenne Peppers and Sauce

Preparation time: 5 minutes | Cooking time: 20 minutes | Servings: 4

Ingredients:

- 1 pound mixed bell peppers, cut into wedges
- ½ cup chicken stock
- ½ cup heavy cream
- A pinch of cayenne pepper
- A pinch of salt and black pepper
- 1 tablespoon cilantro, chopped

Directions:

In your instant pot, combine the bell peppers with the stock and the rest of the ingredients, put the lid on and cook on High for 15 minutes. Release the pressure fast for 5 minutes, divide the mix between plates and serve.

Nutrition: calories 63, fat 5.7, fiber 0.4, carbs 2.8, protein 0.7

Bell Peppers and Brussels Sprouts

Preparation time: 5 minutes | Cooking time: 15 minutes | Servings: 4

Ingredients:

- 1 pound mixed bell peppers, cut into wedges
- ½ pound Brussels sprouts, halved
- 1 cup veggie stock
- 1 tablespoon ghee, melted
- 1 teaspoon smoked paprika
- 1 teaspoon cumin, ground
- 1 tablespoon chives, chopped

Directions:

Set the instant pot on Sauté mode, add the ghee, heat it up, add the peppers and the sprouts and cook for 3 minutes. Put the lid on, cook on High for 12 minutes, release the pressure fast for 5 minutes, divide the mix between plates and serve.

Nutrition: calories 68, fat 4.2, fiber 2.3, carbs 3.4, protein 2.4

Bell Peppers and Mustard Greens
Preparation time: 5 minutes | Cooking time: 20 minutes | Servings: 4

Ingredients:

- 1 pound mixed bell peppers, cut into wedges
- ½ pound mustard greens
- A pinch of salt and black pepper
- 1 cup chicken stock
- 1 tablespoon sweet paprika
- 1 teaspoon chives, chopped

Directions:

In your instant pot, combine the bell peppers with the rest of the ingredients, put the lid on and cook on High for 20 minutes. Release the pressure naturally for 5 minutes, divide the mix between plates and serve.

Nutrition: calories 32, fat 3.4, fiber 2.3, carbs 2.9, protein 2.3

Parmesan Radish
Preparation time: 10 minutes | Cooking time: 10 minutes | Servings: 4

Ingredients:

- 1 pound radishes, sliced
- Juice of 1 lemon
- 1 teaspoon chili powder
- A pinch of salt and black pepper
- 1 cup chicken stock
- 3 tablespoons parmesan, grated

Directions:

In your instant pot, combine the radishes with the lemon juice and the rest of the ingredients, put the lid on and cook on High for 10 minutes. Release the pressure naturally for 10 minutes, divide mix between plates and serve.

Nutrition: calories 38, fat 1.5, fiber 0.2, carbs 0.4, protein 2.5

Cheddar Tomatoes
Preparation time: 10 minutes | Cooking time: 20 minutes | Servings: 4

Ingredients:

- 1 and ½ pounds tomatoes, cut into wedges
- 1 cup cheddar cheese, grated
- 1 cup chicken stock
- A pinch of salt and black pepper
- 1 tablespoon dill, chopped
- 1 teaspoon sweet paprika
- 1 tablespoon chives, chopped

Directions:

In your instant pot, mix tomatoes with the rest of the ingredients except the cheese and toss. Sprinkle the cheese on top, put the lid on and cook on High for 20 minutes. Release the pressure naturally for 10 minutes, divide the mix between plates and serve.

Nutrition: calories 161, fat 10.1, fiber 3.1, carbs 4.5, protein 9.6

Creamy Tomatoes

Preparation time: 10 minutes | Cooking time: 10 minutes | Servings: 4

Ingredients:

- 2 cups cherry tomatoes, halved
- 2 spring onions, chopped
- 1 cup coconut cream
- A pinch of salt and black pepper
- 2 tablespoons garlic, minced
- 1 tablespoon dill, chopped

Directions:

In your instant pot, mix the tomatoes with the spring onions and the rest of the ingredients, put the lid on and cook on High for 10 minutes. Release the pressure naturally for 10 minutes, divide the mix between plates and serve.

Nutrition: calories 165, fat 14.5, fiber 2.8, carbs 6.4, protein 2.7

Garlic Celery and Kale

Preparation time: 10 minutes | Cooking time: 14 minutes | Servings: 4

Ingredients:

- 2 celery stalks, toughly chopped
- 1 pound kale, torn
- 1 tablespoon olive oil
- 4 garlic cloves, minced
- 1 cup chicken stock
- A pinch of salt and black pepper
- 1 tablespoon parsley, chopped

Directions:

Set your instant pot on Sauté mode, add the oil, heat it up, add the garlic and brown for 2 minutes. Add the rest of the ingredients, put the lid on and cook on High for 12 minutes more. Release the pressure naturally for 10 minutes, divide the mix between plates and serve.

Nutrition: calories 95, fat 3.7, fiber 1.9, carbs 2.4, protein 3.8

Creamy Eggplant Mix

Preparation time: 10 minutes | Cooking time: 15 minutes | Servings: 4

Ingredients:

- 2 tablespoons rosemary, chopped
- 2 eggplants, sliced
- A pinch of salt and black pepper
- 1 cup heavy cream
- 1 teaspoon turmeric powder
- 1 tablespoon dill, chopped

Directions:

In your instant pot, mix the eggplants with the rest of the ingredients, put the lid on and cook on High for 15 minutes. Release the pressure naturally for 10 minutes, divide the mix between plates and serve.

Nutrition: calories 181, fat 11.8, fiber 4.2, carbs 5.9, protein 3.6

Spicy Eggplant and Kale Mix

Preparation time: 10 minutes | Cooking time: 15 minutes | Servings: 4

Ingredients:

- 4 small eggplants, sliced
- ¼ cup chicken stock
- 1 tablespoon chili powder
- ½ pound kale, torn
- A pinch of salt and black pepper

Directions:

In your instant pot, mix the eggplants with the stock and the rest of the ingredients, put the lid on and cook on High for 15 minutes. Release the pressure naturally for 10 minutes, divide the mix between plates and serve.

Nutrition: calories 65, fat 1.5, fiber 0.3, carbs 0.9, protein 2.8

Tomato and Dill Sauté

Preparation time: 10 minutes | Cooking time: 15 minutes | Servings: 4

Ingredients:

- 1 pound tomatoes, cubed
- 1 tablespoon dill, chopped
- 1 teaspoon garlic, minced
- A pinch of salt and black pepper
- ½ cup chicken stock
- 1 tablespoon parsley, chopped

Directions:

In your instant pot, mix the tomatoes with the dill and the rest of the ingredients, put the lid on and cook on High for 15 minutes. Release the pressure naturally for 10 minutes, divide the mix between plates and serve.

Nutrition: calories 25, fat 1.9, fiber 0.5, carbs 1.4, protein 1.4

Mustard Greens and Cabbage Sauté

Preparation time: 10 minutes | Cooking time: 15 minutes | Servings: 4

Ingredients:

- 2 cups mustard greens
- 1 red cabbage, shredded
- 1 tablespoon tomato passata
- A pinch of salt and black pepper
- ¼ cup chicken stock
- 1 tablespoon dill, chopped

Directions:

In your instant pot, mix the mustard greens with the cabbage and the rest of the ingredients, put the lid on and cook on High for 15 minutes. Release the pressure naturally for 10 minutes, divide the mix between plates and serve.

Nutrition: calories 36, fat 1.4, fiber 0.2, carbs 0.4, protein 2

Dill Zucchini, Tomatoes and Eggplants

Preparation time: 10 minutes | Cooking time: 15 minutes | Servings: 4

Ingredients:

- 2 cups zucchinis, sliced
- 1 cup tomatoes, cubed
- 1 cup eggplants, sliced
- A pinch of salt and black pepper
- 1 cup tomato passata
- 2 tablespoon dill, chopped

Directions:

In your instant pot, mix the zucchinis with the tomatoes and the rest of the ingredients, put the lid on and cook on High for 15 minutes. Release the pressure naturally for 10 minutes, divide the mix between plates and serve.

Nutrition: calories 41, fat 1.2, fiber 0.2, carbs 0.6, protein 2.4

Balsamic Okra

Preparation time: 10 minutes | Cooking time: 15 minutes | Servings: 4

Ingredients:

- 2 cups okra
- 2 spring onions, chopped
- ½ cup chicken stock
- A pinch of salt and black pepper
- 1 tablespoon balsamic vinegar
- 1 tablespoon dill, chopped

Directions:

In your instant pot, mix the okra with the spring onions and the rest of the ingredients, put the lid on and cook on High for 15 minutes. Release the pressure naturally for 10 minutes, divide the mix between plates and serve.

Nutrition: calories 26, fat 1.2, fiber 0.2, carbs 0.7, protein 1.4

Creamy Okra and Collard Greens

Preparation time: 10 minutes | Cooking time: 20 minutes | Servings: 4

Ingredients:

- 1 pound collard greens, trimmed
- 1 cup okra
- 1 cup heavy cream
- ½ cup chicken stock
- 1 tablespoon sweet paprika
- A pinch of salt and black pepper
- 1 tablespoon cilantro, chopped

Directions:

In your instant pot, combine the collard greens with the okra and the rest of the ingredients, put the lid on and cook on High for 20 minutes. Release the pressure naturally for 10 minutes, divide the mix between plates and serve.

Nutrition: calories 151, fat 12.2, fiber 4.3, carbs 6.8, protein 4

Balsamic Savoy Cabbage

Preparation time: 10 minutes | Cooking time: 20 minutes | Servings: 4

Ingredients:

- 1 Savoy cabbage, shredded
- ½ cup chicken stock
- 1 tablespoon dill, chopped
- A pinch of salt and black pepper
- 1 tablespoon balsamic vinegar

Directions:

In your instant pot, mix the Savoy cabbage with the chicken stock and the rest of the ingredients, put the lid on and cook on High for 20 minutes. Release the pressure naturally for 10 minutes, divide the mix between plates and serve.

Nutrition: calories 61, fat 1.3, fiber 0.8, carbs 1, protein 3.2

Cilantro Red Cabbage and Artichokes

Preparation time: 10 minutes | Cooking time: 20 minutes | Servings: 4

Ingredients:

- ½ cup canned artichoke hearts, drained and chopped
- 3 garlic cloves, minced
- 2 small red cabbage heads, shredded
- A pinch of salt and black pepper
- 1 cup chicken stock
- ½ cup tomato passata
- 1 tablespoon cilantro, chopped

Directions:

In your instant pot, combine the artichokes with the garlic and the rest of the ingredients except the cilantro, put the lid on and cook on High for 20 minutes. Release the pressure naturally for 10 minutes, divide the mix between plates and serve with the cilantro sprinkled on top.

Nutrition: calories 141, fat 1.5, fiber 0.2, carbs 1.2, protein 7.3

Dill Fennel and Brussels Sprouts

Preparation time: 10 minutes | Cooking time: 15 minutes | Servings: 4

Ingredients:

- 2 fennel bulbs, cut into wedges
- 1 pound Brussels sprouts, halved
- A pinch of salt and black pepper
- 1 cup chicken stock
- 1 tablespoon dill, chopped
- ¼ cup tomato passata

Directions:

In your instant pot, mix the fennel with the sprouts and the rest of the ingredients, put the lid on and cook on High for 15 minutes. Release the pressure naturally for 10 minutes, divide the mix between plates and serve.

Nutrition: calories 96, fat 1.4, fiber 0.8, carbs 1, protein 5.6

Cinnamon Green Beans Mix

Preparation time: 10 minutes | Cooking time: 15 minutes | Servings: 4

Ingredients:

- 1 pound green beans, trimmed
- A pinch of salt and black pepper
- ½ cup chicken stock
- 1 teaspoon chili powder
- 1 tablespoon rosemary, chopped
- ½ teaspoon cinnamon powder

Directions:

In your instant pot, combine the green beans with the stock and the rest of the ingredients, put the lid on and cook on High for 15 minutes. Release the pressure naturally for 10 minutes, divide the mix between plates and serve.

Nutrition: calories 41, fat 1.4, fiber 0.1, carbs 0.5, protein 2.3

Okra and Olives Mix

Preparation time: 10 minutes | Cooking time: 15 minutes | Servings: 4

Ingredients:

- 2 cups okra
- 1 cup kalamata olives, pitted and sliced
- A pinch of salt and black pepper
- Juice of ½ lime
- ½ cup veggie stock
- 2 tablespoons tomato passata
- 2 tablespoons parsley, chopped

Directions:

In your instant pot, mix the okra with the olives and the rest of the ingredients, put the lid on and cook on High for 15 minutes. Release the pressure naturally for 10 minutes, divide the mix between plates and serve.

Nutrition: calories 64, fat 4, fiber 2.8, carbs 3, protein 1.4

Olives, Capers and Kale

Preparation time: 10 minutes | Cooking time: 20 minutes | Servings: 4

Ingredients:

- 1 cup black olives, pitted and sliced
- 2 spring onions, chopped
- 1 tablespoon capers, drained
- ½ cup chicken stock
- 1 pound kale, torn
- A pinch of salt and black pepper
- 1 tablespoon parsley, chopped

Directions:

In your instant pot, combine kale with the olives, capers and the rest of the ingredients, put the lid on and cook on High for 20 minutes. Release the pressure naturally for 10 minutes, divide the mix between plates and serve.

Nutrition: calories 99, fat 3.7, fiber 2.3, carbs 3, protein 4

Eggplants and Cabbage Mix

Preparation time: 5 minutes | Cooking time: 15 minutes | Servings: 4

Ingredients:

- 1 big eggplant, peeled and sliced
- 2 garlic cloves, minced
- A pinch of salt and black pepper
- 1 green cabbage, shredded
- 1 cup chicken stock
- 1 tablespoon dill, chopped
- 1 teaspoon cumin, ground

Directions:

In your instant pot, mix the eggplant with the garlic, cabbage and the rest of the ingredients, put the lid on and cook on High for 15 minutes. Release the pressure fast for 5 minutes, divide the mix between plates and serve.

Nutrition: calories 94, fat 1.5, fiber 0.4, carbs 1, protein 4.5

Eggplants, Cucumber and Olives

Preparation time: 10 minutes | Cooking time: 12 minutes | Servings: 4

Ingredients:

- 2 and ½ cups eggplant, sliced
- 1 tablespoon avocado oil
- 2 cucumbers, cubed
- 1 shallot, minced
- 1 cup black olives, pitted and sliced
- A pinch of salt and black pepper
- ½ cup chicken stock

Directions:

Set the instant pot on Sauté mode, add the oil, heat it up, add the shallot and cook for 2 minutes. Add the eggplant and the rest of the ingredients, put the lid on and cook on High for 10 minutes. Release the pressure naturally for 10 minutes, divide the mix between plates and serve.

Nutrition: calories 83, fat 4.4, fiber 2.3, carbs 3.4, protein 2

Lemon Peppers and Bok Choy

Preparation time: 10 minutes | Cooking time: 20 minutes | Servings: 4

Ingredients:

- 1 pound mixed bell peppers, cut into wedges
- 1 cup bok choy, chopped
- 2 tablespoons sweet paprika
- A pinch of salt and black pepper
- ½ cup chicken stock
- ¼ cup lemon juice
- 1 tablespoon cilantro, chopped

Directions:

In your instant pot, mix the bell peppers with the bok choy and the rest of the ingredients except the cilantro, put the lid on and cook on High for 20 minutes. Release the pressure naturally for 10 minutes, divide the mix between plates, sprinkle the cilantro on top and serve.

Nutrition: calories 34, fat 1, fiber 0.2, carbs 0.5, protein 1.3

Tomato Bok Choy Mix

Preparation time: 10 minutes | Cooking time: 15 minutes | Servings: 4

Ingredients:

- 1 pound bok choy, torn
- 1 cup cherry tomatoes, halved
- 2 tablespoons lime juice
- ½ cup chicken stock
- 1 tablespoon ginger, grated
- 1 tablespoon chives, chopped
- 1 tablespoon oregano, chopped
- 1 tablespoon olive oil

Directions:

Set the instant pot on Sauté mode, add the oil, heat it up, add the ginger and sauté for 2 minutes. Add the rest of the ingredients, put the lid on and cook on High for 12 minutes. Release the pressure naturally for 10 minutes, divide the mix between plates and serve.

Nutrition: calories 62, fat 4.1, fiber 2.3, carbs 3, protein 2.5

Garlic Cabbage and Watercress

Preparation time: 10 minutes | Cooking time: 16 minutes | Servings: 4

Ingredients:

- 1 pound red cabbage, shredded
- 2 garlic cloves, chopped
- 1 tablespoon ghee, melted
- 1 cup chicken stock
- 1 bunch watercress, trimmed
- 1 tablespoon cilantro, chopped

Directions:

Set your instant pot on Sauté mode, add the ghee, heat it up, add the garlic, stir and cook for 2 minutes. Add the cabbage and the rest of the ingredients, put the lid on and cook on High for 14 minutes. Release the pressure naturally for 10 minutes, divide the mix between plates and serve.

Nutrition: calories 63, fat 3.5, fiber 2, carbs 3.1, protein 2

Mint and Basil Eggplant

Preparation time: 10 minutes | Cooking time: 20 minutes | Servings: 4

Ingredients:

- 1 pound eggplants cubed
- 2 spring onions, chopped
- 1 cup chicken stock
- 1 tablespoon olive oil
- 1 tablespoon mint, chopped
- 1 tablespoon basil, chopped
- 1 teaspoon sweet paprika
- A pinch of salt and black pepper

Directions:

Set your instant pot on Sauté mode, add the oil, heat it up, add the onions and sauté for 2 minutes. Add the eggplants and the rest of the ingredients, put the lid on and cook on High for 18 minutes. Release the pressure naturally for 10 minutes, divide the mix into bowls and serve.

Nutrition: calories 76, fat 3.7, fiber 0.5, carbs 1.2, protein 0.5

Broccoli and Watercress Mix

Preparation time: 10 minutes | Cooking time: 15 minutes | Servings: 4

Ingredients:

- 1 pound broccoli florets
- 1 tablespoon olive oil
- 2 shallots, chopped
- 1 bunch watercress
- 1 tablespoon sweet paprika
- ½ cup tomato passata

Directions:

Set the instant pot on Sauté mode, add the oil, heat it up, add the shallots and cook for 2 minutes Add the rest of the ingredients, put the lid on and cook on High for 13 minutes. Release the pressure naturally for 10 minutes, divide the mix into bowls and serve.

Nutrition: calories 81, fat 4.2, fiber 2.3, carbs 3.5, protein 3.8

Balsamic Bok Choy and Onions

Preparation time: 10 minutes | Cooking time: 20 minutes | Servings: 4

Ingredients:

- 1 pound bok choy, torn
- 2 spring onions, chopped
- 1 cup chicken stock
- 4 garlic cloves, chopped
- 1 tablespoon balsamic vinegar
- A pinch of salt and black pepper
- ¼ teaspoon red pepper flakes
- 1 tablespoon dill, chopped

Directions:

In your instant pot, combine the bok choy with the spring onions and the rest of the ingredients, put the lid on and cook on High for 20 minutes. Release the pressure naturally for 10 minutes, divide the mix between plates and serve.

Nutrition: calories 34, fat 1.2, fiber 0.4, carbs 0.4, protein 2.5

Balsamic and Coconut Cabbage

Preparation time: 10 minutes | Cooking time: 14 minutes | Servings: 4

Ingredients:

- ½ cup veggie stock
- 1 pound red cabbage, cut into wedges
- ½ cup coconut aminos
- 2 tablespoons balsamic vinegar
- 1 teaspoon thyme, dried
- A pinch of salt and black pepper
- 2 tablespoons ghee, melted

Directions:

Set the instant pot on Sauté mode, add ghee, heat it up, add the cabbage and sauté for 2 minutes. Add the rest of the ingredients, put the lid on and cook on High for 12 minutes. Release the pressure naturally for 10 minutes, divide the mix between plates and serve.

Nutrition: calories 118, fat 6.8, fiber 2.9, carbs 5.1, protein 1.5

Buttery Turmeric Brussels Sprouts

Preparation time: 10 minutes | Cooking time: 10 minutes | Servings: 4

Ingredients:

- 2 pounds Brussels sprouts, halved
- A pinch of salt and black pepper
- 2 tablespoons ghee, melted
- 2 teaspoons turmeric powder
- 1 teaspoon lime zest, grated
- ¼ cup chicken stock
- 2 tablespoons coconut aminos

Directions:

Set the instant pot on Sauté mode, add the ghee, heat it up, add the sprouts and turmeric and coo for 2 minutes. Add the rest of the ingredients, put the lid on and cook on High for 8 minutes. Release the pressure naturally for 10 minutes, divide the mix between plates and serve.

Nutrition: calories 166, fat 7.3, fiber 3.4, carbs 4.4, protein 7.8

Lemon and Pesto Broccoli

Preparation time: 5 minutes | Cooking time: 15 minutes | Servings: 4

Ingredients:

- 1 and ½ pounds broccoli florets
- 1 tablespoon lemon juice
- 1 tablespoon lemon zest, grated
- 1 tablespoon basil pesto
- ½ cup chicken stock
- A pinch of salt and black pepper

Directions:

In your instant pot, mix the broccoli with the lemon juice and the rest of the ingredients, put the lid on and cook on High for 15 minutes. Release the pressure fast for 5 minutes, divide the mix between plates and serve.

Nutrition: calories 81, fat 1.2, fiber 0.5, carbs 1, protein 6.5

Bok Choy and Parmesan Mix

Preparation time: 5 minutes | Cooking time: 10 minutes | Servings: 4

Ingredients:

- 2 cups bok choy, torn
- ½ cup chicken stock
- 2 tablespoons dill, chopped
- 1 tablespoon tomato passata
- 3 tablespoons parmesan cheese, grated

Directions:

In your instant pot, combine the bok choy with the stock and the other ingredients except the parmesan, put the lid on and cook on High for 10 minutes. Release the pressure fast for 5 minutes, divide the mix between plates, sprinkle the parmesan on top and serve.

Nutrition: calories 24, fat 1.6, fiber 0.6, carbs 1, protein 2.5

Milky Fennel

Preparation time: 5 minutes | Cooking time: 12 minutes | Servings: 4

Ingredients:

- 2 big fennel bulbs, sliced
- 2 tablespoons ghee, melted
- 2 cups almond milk
- ½ teaspoon nutmeg, ground
- A pinch of salt and black pepper

Directions:

In your instant pot, combine the fennel with the melted ghee and the rest of the ingredients, put the lid on and cook on High for 12 minutes. Release the pressure fast for 5 minutes, divide the mix between plates and serve.

Nutrition: calories 243, fat 20.4, fiber 4.3, carbs 5.7, protein 4.2

Minty Green Beans

Preparation time: 10 minutes | Cooking time: 15 minutes | Servings: 4

Ingredients:

- 1 pound green beans, trimmed
- 1 green onion, sliced
- 1 tablespoon mint, chopped
- 1 cup chicken stock
- A pinch of salt and black pepper
- 1 tablespoon cilantro, chopped

Directions:

In your instant pot, combine the green beans with the green onion and the rest of the ingredients, put the lid on and cook on High for 15 minutes. Release the pressure naturally for 10 minutes, divide the mix between plates and serve.

Nutrition: calories 40, fat 1.2, fiber 0.4, carbs 0.6, protein 2.4

Almonds Green Beans Mix

Preparation time: 10 minutes | Cooking time: 15 minutes | Servings: 4

Ingredients:

- 1 pound green beans, trimmed
- 1 tablespoon balsamic vinegar
- A pinch of salt and black pepper
- 2 tablespoons almonds, chopped
- 1 tablespoon dill, chopped
- ½ cup chicken stock

Directions:

In your instant pot, combine the green beans with the vinegar, almonds and the rest of the ingredients, put the lid on and cook on High for 15 minutes. Release the pressure naturally for 10 minutes, divide the mix between plates and serve.

Nutrition: calories 56, fat 1.7, fiber 0.5, carbs 1, protein 2.9

Mixed Peppers and Parsley

Preparation time: 10 minutes | Cooking time: 12 minutes | Servings: 4

Ingredients:

- 1 yellow bell pepper, cut into wedges
- 1 green bell pepper, cut into wedges
- 2 red bell peppers, cut into wedges
- 2 garlic cloves, minced
- A pinch of salt and black pepper
- ½ cup chicken stock
- 1 bunch parsley, chopped

Directions:

In your instant pot, combine the bell peppers with the garlic and the rest of the ingredients, put the lid on and cook on High for 12 minutes. Release the pressure naturally for 10 minutes, divide the mix between plates and serve.

Nutrition: calories 25, fat 1, fiber 0.1, carbs 0.5, protein 1

Peppers, Green Beans and Olives Mix

Preparation time: 10 minutes | Cooking time: 15 minutes | Servings: 4

Ingredients:

- 2 red bell peppers, cut into wedges
- A pinch of salt and black pepper
- 2 garlic cloves, minced
- ½ cup chicken stock
- ¼ pound green beans, trimmed and halved
- 1 cup black olives

Directions:

In your instant pot, combine the bell peppers with the other ingredients, put the lid on and cook on High for 15 minutes. Release the pressure naturally for 10 minutes, divide the mix between plates and serve.

Nutrition: calories 70, fat 3.9, fiber 2.8, carbs 3.2, protein 1.6

Lemon Tomato and Green Beans

Preparation time: 10 minutes | Cooking time: 15 minutes | Servings: 4

Ingredients:

- 1 and ½ pounds green beans, trimmed
- A pinch of salt and black pepper
- 14 ounces canned tomatoes, crushed
- 1 bunch parsley, chopped
- 2 garlic cloves, crushed
- 1 cup chicken stock
- Juice of 1 lemon
- A pinch of red pepper flakes

Directions:

In your instant pot, combine the green beans with the tomatoes and the rest of the ingredients, put the lid on and cook on High for 15 minutes. Release the pressure naturally for 10 minutes, divide the mix between plates and serve.

Nutrition: calories 94, fat 1.4, fiber 0.2, carbs 0.6, protein 5.3

Ketogenic Instant Pot Dessert Recipes

Sweet Zucchini Pudding
Preparation time: 10 minutes | Cooking time: 40 minutes | Servings: 4

Ingredients:
- 3 cups zucchinis, grated
- 1 cup swerve
- 1 tablespoon vanilla extract
- 2 eggs, whisked
- 1 cup coconut flour
- Cooking spray
- 1 cup water

Directions:
In a bowl mix the zucchinis with the rest of the ingredients except the water and the cooking spray and whisk well. Grease a pudding pan that fits the instant pot with the cooking spray and pour the zucchini mix inside. Add the water to the instant pot, add the steamer basket, put the pan, put the lid on and cook on High for 40 minutes. Release the pressure naturally for 10 minutes and serve the pudding cold.

Nutrition: calories 176, fat 5.5, fiber 3.4, carbs 4.6, protein 7.8

Almond Strawberry Bread
Preparation time: 5 minutes | Cooking time: 40 minutes | Servings: 6

Ingredients:
- ¾ cup swerve
- 1/3 cup ghee, melted
- 1 teaspoon vanilla extract
- 2 eggs, whisked
- 2 cups strawberries
- 1 teaspoon baking powder
- 1 and ½ cups almond milk
- 1/3 cup almond flour
- 2 cups water
- Cooking spray

Directions:
In a bowl, mix the ghee with the strawberries and the rest of the ingredients except the cooking spray and the water and whisk well. Grease a loaf pan that fits the instant pot with the cooking spray and pour the mix inside. Add the water to your instant pot, add the steamer basket, add the loaf pan inside, put the lid on and cook on High for 40 minutes. Release the pressure fast for 5 minutes, cool the bread, slice and serve.

Nutrition: calories 361, fat 18.2, fiber 3.4, carbs 5.9, protein 5.9

Coconut Zucchini Cake

Preparation time: 10 minutes | Cooking time: 40 minutes | Servings: 4

Ingredients:

- 2 egg, whisked
- ½ cup swerve
- 2 tablespoons ghee, melted
- 1 cup coconut milk
- ¼ cup coconut flour
- 2 zucchinis, grated
- ½ teaspoon baking soda
- Cooking spray
- 2 cups water

Directions:

In a bowl, mix the eggs with the zucchinis and the rest of the ingredients except the water and the cooking spray and whisk well. Grease a cake pan with the cooking spray and pour the zucchini mix inside. Add the water to the pot, add steamer basket, add the cake pan inside, put the lid on and cook on High for 40 minutes. Release the pressure naturally for 10 minutes, cool the cake, slice and serve.

Nutrition: calories 242, fat 23.2, fiber 2.4, carbs 6.8, protein 5.4

Vanilla Blackberries Bowls

Preparation time: 10 minutes | Cooking time: 10 minutes | Servings: 4

Ingredients:

- 2 teaspoons vanilla extract
- 3 cups blackberries
- 1 tablespoon swerve
- ½ cup coconut nectar

Directions:

In your instant pot, mix the blackberries with the vanilla and the rest of the ingredients, put the lid on and cook on High for 10 minutes. Release the pressure naturally for 10 minutes, divide the mix into bowls and serve.

Nutrition: calories 70, fat 1, fiber 0.4, carbs 0.9, protein 1.6

Plums and Raisins Mix

Preparation time: 10 minutes | Cooking time: 15 minutes | Servings: 4

Ingredients:

- 1 pound plums, pitted and halved
- 1 cup coconut water
- ¼ cup raisins
- ½ cup swerve
- 1 teaspoon vanilla extract

Directions:

In your instant pot, combine the plums with the water and the rest of the ingredients, put the lid on and cook on High for 15 minutes. Release the pressure naturally for 10 minutes, divide the mix into bowls and serve.

Nutrition: calories 50, fat 1.2, fiber 0.1, carbs 0.6, protein 0.8

Berry Chocolate Cream

Preparation time: 5 minutes | Cooking time: 10 minutes | Servings: 4

Ingredients:

- 2 cups heavy cream
- 4 ounces chocolate, cut into chunks and melted
- 1 teaspoon stevia
- 1 cup blackberries
- 2 cups water

Directions:

In a bowl, mix the heavy cream with the chocolate and the rest of the ingredients except the water, whisk well and divide into ramekins. Put the water in your instant pot, add the steamer basket, add the ramekins inside, put the lid on and cook on High for 10 minutes. Release the pressure fast for 5 minutes, and serve the cream cold.

Nutrition: calories 360, fat 17.2, fiber 2.9, carbs 6.4, protein 3.9

Strawberries and Pecans Cream

Preparation time: 10 minutes | Cooking time: 10 minutes | Servings: 4

Ingredients:

- 4 ounces strawberries
- 4 ounces coconut cream
- 1 cup stevia
- 1 teaspoon vanilla extract
- 2 tablespoons pecans, chopped
- 1 and ½ cups water

Directions:

In a bowl, mix the strawberries with the cream and the other ingredients except the water, whisk well and divide into 4 ramekins. Add the water to your instant pot, add the steamer basket, add the ramekins inside, put the lid on and cook on High for 10 minutes. Release the pressure naturally for 10 minutes, and serve cold.

Nutrition: calories 129, fat 11.8, fiber 2.3, carbs 5.1, protein 1.6

Coconut and Macadamia Chocolate Cream

Preparation time: 10 minutes | Cooking time: 15 minutes | Serving: 4

Ingredients:

- 3 ounces chocolate, unsweetened and melted
- 2 tablespoons macadamia nuts, chopped
- 2 tablespoons coconut, unsweetened and shredded
- 2 eggs, whisked
- 1 cup coconut cream
- ¾ cup swerve
- 2 cups water

Directions:

In a bowl, mix the chocolate with the nuts and the other ingredients except the water, whisk well and divide into ramekins. Add the water to the instant pot, add the steamer basket, put the ramekins inside, put the lid on and cook on High for 15 minutes. Release the pressure naturally for 10 minutes and serve the cream cold.

Nutrition: calories 300, fat 15.8, fiber 2.6, carbs 5.8, protein 6.2

Cantaloupe Pudding

Preparation time: 10 minutes | Cooking time: 15 minutes | Servings: 4

Ingredients:

- 2 and ½ cups coconut milk
- 1 cup coconut cream
- ½ cup swerve
- 1 teaspoon vanilla extract
- 1 egg, whisked
- 1 teaspoon baking powder
- 2 cups cantaloupe, cubed
- 2 cups water

Directions:

In a bowl, combine the coconut milk with the cream and the other ingredients except the water, whisk well and pour into a pudding pan. Put the water in the instant pot, add the steamer basket, put the pan inside, put the lid on and cook on High for 15 minutes. Release the pressure naturally for 10 minutes, divide the pudding into bowls and serve.

Nutrition: calories 184, fat 15.6, fiber 2.1, carbs 7.5, protein 3.4

Coconut Raspberries Bowls

Preparation time: 10 minutes | Cooking time: 25 minutes | Servings: 4

Ingredients:

- 1 cup coconut, unsweetened and shredded
- 2 eggs, whisked
- 1 cup coconut milk
- ¾ cup swerve
- 1 teaspoon vanilla extract
- 1 cup raspberries

Directions:

In your instant pot, mix the coconut with the eggs and the rest of the ingredients, whisk well, put the lid on and cook on Low for 25 minutes. Release the pressure naturally for 10 minutes, divide the mix into bowls and serve.

Nutrition: calories 259, fat 22.3, fiber 3.5, carbs 6.8, protein 5.3

Watermelon Cream

Preparation time: 10 minutes | Cooking time: 10 minutes | Servings: 4

Ingredients:

- 2 cups watermelon, peeled and cubed
- 1 cup heavy cream
- 1 tablespoon vanilla extract
- ½ cup swerve
- 1 cup water

Directions:

In a bowl, mix the watermelon and the cream and the other ingredients except the water, whisk and divide into 4 ramekins. Add the water to the instant pot, add the steamer basket, put the ramekins inside, put the lid on and cook on High for 10 minutes. Release the pressure naturally for 10 minutes and serve the mix cold.

Nutrition: calories 136, fat 11.2, fiber 0.2, carbs 7, protein 1.1

Lemon Strawberries Stew

Preparation time: 10 minutes | Cooking time: 20 minutes | Servings: 4

Ingredients:

- 3 cups strawberries
- 1 tablespoon lemon zest, grated
- 1 tablespoon lemon juice
- 1 cup swerve
- 1 teaspoon vanilla extract
- 1 cup water

Directions:

In your instant pot, combine the strawberries with the lemon zest and the rest of the ingredients, put the lid on and cook on High for 20 minutes. Release the pressure naturally for 10 minutes, divide the mix into bowls and serve right away.

Nutrition: calories 82, fat 1.4, fiber 0.5, carbs 1, protein 0.8

Egg and Cantaloupe Pudding

Preparation time: 10 minutes | Cooking time: 25 minutes | Servings: 4

Ingredients:

- 4 eggs, whisked
- 1 teaspoon baking soda
- 2 cups heavy cream
- 1 cantaloupe, peeled and cubed
- ½ teaspoon vanilla extract
- 1 cup swerve
- 2 cups water

Directions:

In a bowl mix the eggs with the cream and the rest of the ingredients except the water, whisk well and pour into a pudding pan. Add the water to the pot, add the steamer basket, add the pudding pan inside, put the lid on and cook on High for 25 minutes. Release the pressure naturally for 10 minutes, and serve the pudding cold.

Nutrition: calories 283, fat 11.8, fiber 0.3, carbs 4.7, protein 7.1

Cocoa Strawberries Mix

Preparation time: 10 minutes | Cooking time: 15 minutes | Servings: 4

Ingredients:

- 2 cups strawberries
- 1 teaspoon vanilla extract
- 1 tablespoon cocoa powder
- 2 cups coconut water
- 2 tablespoons swerve

Directions:

In your instant pot, mix the strawberries with the vanilla and the rest of the ingredients, put the lid on and cook on High for 15 minutes. Release the pressure naturally for 10 minutes, divide the mix into bowls and serve.

Nutrition: calories 72, fat 1.8, fiber 0.2, carbs 0.7, protein 1.6

Lime Cherry Bowls

Preparation time: 10 minutes | Cooking time: 10 minutes | Servings: 4

Ingredients:

- ½ cup cherries, pitted
- Juice of 1 lime
- Zest of 1 lime, grated
- 1 cup coconut water
- ½ cup coconut, unsweetened and shredded
- ½ teaspoon vanilla extract

Directions:

In your instant pot, mix the cherries with the lime juice and the rest of the ingredients, put the lid on and cook on High for 10 minutes. Release the pressure naturally for 10 minutes, divide the mix into bowls and serve cold.

Nutrition: calories 72, fat 3.4, fiber 1, carbs 1.5, protein 0.5

Zucchini Rice Pudding

Preparation time: 10 minutes | Cooking time: 20 minutes | Servings: 4

Ingredients:

- 2 cups cauliflower rice
- 1 cup zucchinis, grated
- 3 cups coconut milk
- 3 tablespoon swerve
- 1 teaspoon vanilla extract
- 1 tablespoon cinnamon powder

Directions:

In your instant pot, mix the cauliflower rice with the zucchinis and the rest of the ingredients, put the lid on and cook on High for 20 minutes. Release the pressure naturally for 10 minutes, divide the rice into bowls and serve.

Nutrition: calories 122, fat 12.3, fiber 3.1, carbs 4.6, protein 4.5

Creamy Rice Pudding

Preparation time: 10 minutes | Cooking time: 20 minutes | Servings: 4

Ingredients:

- 2 cups cream cheese, soft
- 2 cups heavy cream
- 3 tablespoons swerve
- 2 cups cauliflower rice
- 1 teaspoon lemon zest, grated
- 1 cup water

Directions:

In a bowl, whisk the cream with the cream cheese and the rest of the ingredients except the water, whisk really well and divide into 4 ramekins. Put the water in your instant pot, add the steamer basket, put the ramekins inside, put the lid on and cook on High for 20 minutes. Release the pressure naturally for 10 minutes and serve the puddings warm.

Nutrition: calories 306, fat 13.4, fiber 0, carbs 2.4, protein 5

Berries and Nuts Pudding

Preparation time: 10 minutes | Cooking time: 20 minutes | Servings: 4

Ingredients:

- 1 cup blackberries
- ½ cup blueberries
- 1 egg, whisked
- 1 teaspoon baking soda
- 2 cups coconut milk
- 1 tablespoon macadamia nuts, chopped
- 1 tablespoon pecans, chopped
- 3 tablespoons swerve
- 1 cup coconut cream
- 1 cup water

Directions:

In a bowl, mix the berries with the egg and the rest of the ingredients except the water, whisk well and pour into a pudding pan. Put the water in the instant pot, add the steamer basket, put the pudding pan inside, put the lid on and cook on High for 20 minutes. Release the pressure naturally for 10 minutes and serve the pudding cold.

Nutrition: calories 342, fat 14.8, fiber 3.4, carbs 6.4, protein 6.2

Lime Coconut Vanilla Cream

Preparation time: 10 minutes | Cooking time: 20 minutes | Servings: 4

Ingredients:

- 2 cups coconut cream
- 1 tablespoon lime zest
- 1 tablespoon lime juice
- 4 eggs, whisked
- 2 teaspoon vanilla extract
- 1 cup water

Directions:

In a bowl, combine the coconut cream with the rest of the ingredients except the water, whisk well and divide into 4 ramekins. Put the water in the instant pot, add the steamer basket, put the ramekins inside, put the lid on and cook on High for 20 minutes. Release the pressure naturally for 10 minutes and serve.

Nutrition: calories 342, fat 22.7, fiber 2.7, carbs 7.4, protein 8.3

Plums Jam

Preparation time: 10 minutes | Cooking time: 30 minutes | Servings: 4

Ingredients:

- Juice of 1 lemon
- 1 tablespoon lemon zest, grated
- 1 cup swerve
- 2 cups plums, pitted and halved
- 1 cup water

Directions:

In your instant pot, mix the plums with the rest of the ingredients, put the lid on and cook on Low for 30 minutes. Release the pressure naturally for 10 minutes, blend the mix using an immersion blender, divide into jars and serve.

Nutrition: calories 42, fat 1.7, fiber 0.2, carbs 0.3, protein 0.4

Raspberries and Coconut Puddings

Preparation time: 10 minutes | Cooking time: 25 minutes | Servings: 4

Ingredients:

- 2 cups raspberries
- Zest of 1 lime, grated
- 2 cups coconut cream
- ½ cup coconut, unsweetened and shredded
- 1 teaspoon vanilla extract
- 1 cup water

Directions:

In a bowl, mix the berries with the rest of the ingredients except the water, whisk well and divide into 4 ramekins. Put the water in the instant pot, add the steamer basket, add the ramekins inside, put the lid on and cook on High for 25 minutes. Release the pressure naturally for 10 minutes and serve the puddings cold.

Nutrition: calories 346, fat 15.8, fiber 2.7, carbs 6.5, protein 3.8

Cinnamon Cream

Preparation time: 10 minutes | Cooking time: 20 minutes | Servings: 4

Ingredients:

- 4 eggs, whisked
- 2 tablespoons lime juice
- 1 teaspoon lime zest, grated
- 1 cup swerve
- 1 and ½ cups coconut cream
- 1 tablespoon cinnamon powder
- 1 and ½ cups water

Directions:

In a bowl, mix the eggs with the lime juice and the rest of the ingredients except the water, whisk well and divide into 4 ramekins. Put the water in the instant pot, add the steamer basket, put the ramekins inside, put the lid on and cook on High for 20 minutes. Release the pressure naturally for 10 minutes, and serve the cream cold.

Nutrition: calories 374, fat 22.1, fiber 3.2, carbs 5.9, protein 8.8

Lemon Cantaloupe Stew

Preparation time: 10 minutes | Cooking time: 15 minutes | Servings: 4

Ingredients:

- 2 cups cantaloupe, peeled and cubed
- ½ cup swerve
- 1 cup water
- 1 teaspoon vanilla extract

Directions:

In your instant pot, mix the cantaloupe with the rest of the ingredients, put the lid on and cook on High for 15 minutes. Release the pressure naturally for 10 minutes, divide the stew into bowls and serve.

Nutrition: calories 41, fat 1.7, fiber 0.7, carbs 1, protein 0.8

Ginger Chocolate Cream

Preparation time: 10 minutes | Cooking time: 15 minutes | Servings: 4

Ingredients:

- 4 ounces chocolate, unsweetened and melted
- 2 tablespoons swerve
- 1 tablespoon ginger, grated
- 2 cups coconut cream
- 1 teaspoon vanilla extract
- 1 cup water

Directions:

In a bowl, mix the chocolate with the sugar, ginger and the rest of the ingredients except the water, whisk and divide into 4 ramekins. Put the water in the instant pot, add the steamer basket, put the ramekins inside, put the lid on and cook on High for 15 minutes. Release the pressure naturally for 10 minutes, and serve the cream cold.

Nutrition: calories 235, fat 14.1, fiber 3.8, carbs 4.1, protein 5

Macadamia Blackberry Stew

Preparation time: 5 minutes | Cooking time: 20 minutes | Servings: 4

Ingredients:

- 12 ounces blackberries
- 2 tablespoons lime juice
- 2 tablespoons stevia
- 1 and ½ cups coconut nectar
- 1 tablespoon macadamia nuts, chopped
- 1 teaspoon vanilla extract

Directions:

In your instant pot, mix the blackberries with the rest of the ingredients, put the lid on and cook on High for 15 minutes. Release the pressure fast for 5 minutes, divide the mix into bowls and serve.

Nutrition: calories 78, fat 2, fiber 1.2, carbs 1.5, protein 1.4

Plums and Berries Compote

Preparation time: 10 minutes | Cooking time: 20 minutes | Servings: 4

Ingredients:

- 1 cup plums, pitted and halved
- 1 cup blueberries
- 2 tablespoons lemon juice
- 1 and ½ cups water
- ¾ cup swerve
- 1 teaspoon vanilla extract

Directions:

In your instant pot, mix the plums with the berries and the rest of the ingredients, put the lid on and cook on High for 20 minutes. Release the pressure naturally for 10 minutes, divide the compote into bowls and serve.

Nutrition: calories 43, fat 1.2, fiber 0.1, carbs 1, protein 0.5

Lime Watermelon Compote

Preparation time: 5 minutes | *Cooking time: 10 minutes* | *Servings: 4*

Ingredients:

- 1 and ½ cups watermelon, peeled and cubed
- 2 tablespoons lime juice
- 2 cups water
- 3 tablespoons swerve

Directions:

In your instant pot, mix the watermelon with the rest of the ingredients, put the lid on and cook on High for 10 minutes. Release the pressure fast for 5 minutes, divide the mix into bowls and serve really cold.

Nutrition: calories 40, fat 1, fiber 0.1, carbs 0.2, protein 0.6

Heavy Cream and Raspberries Ramekins

Preparation time: 5 minutes | *Cooking time: 8 minutes* | *Servings: 4*

Ingredients:

- 2 cups raspberries
- 1 cup heavy cream
- ¼ cup swerve
- 2 tablespoons ghee, melted
- 1 teaspoon vanilla extract
- ½ teaspoon ginger powder
- 1 cup water

Directions:

In a bowl, mix the raspberries with the cream and the rest of the ingredients except the water, whisk and divide into ramekins. Put the water in the instant pot, add the steamer basket, put the ramekins inside, put the lid on and cook on High for 8 minutes. Release the pressure fast for 5 minutes, and serve cold.

Nutrition: calories 195, fat 17.9, fiber 4, carbs 7.5, protein 1.4

Coconut Pecans Cream

Preparation time: 10 minutes | *Cooking time: 15 minutes* | *Servings: 4*

Ingredients:

- 1 cup pecans, chopped
- 1 cup coconut cream
- ½ cup coconut, unsweetened and shredded
- 4 tablespoons swerve
- 1 teaspoon vanilla extract
- 1 cup water

Directions:

In a bowl, mix the pecans with the rest of the ingredients except the water, whisk and divide into ramekins. Put the water in the instant pot, add the steamer basket inside, add the ramekins, put the lid on and cook on High for 15 minutes. Release the pressure naturally for 10 minutes and serve cold.

Nutrition: calories 176, fat 17.6, fiber 2.2, carbs 5, protein 1.7

Chocolate and Brazil Nuts Bread

Preparation time: 10 minutes | Cooking time: 30 minutes | Servings: 4

Ingredients:

- 1 cup coconut milk
- 2 eggs, whisked
- 2 teaspoons vanilla extract
- 1 cup swerve
- 1 cup brazil nuts, peeled and chopped
- 2 cups coconut flour
- 2 ounces chocolate, melted
- ¼ teaspoon baking powder
- 2 cups water
- Cooking spray

Directions:

In a bowl, combine the coconut milk with the eggs and the rest of the ingredients except the cooking spray and the water and whisk well. Grease a loaf pan with the cooking spray and pour the bread mix inside. Add the water to the instant pot, add the steamer basket, put the loaf pan inside, put the lid on and cook on High for 30 minutes. Release the pressure naturally for 10 minutes, cool the bread down and serve.

Nutrition: calories 253, fat 19.7, fiber 1.8, carbs 6.8, protein 5.2

Greek Pudding

Preparation time: 10 minutes | Cooking time: 30 minutes | Servings: 4

Ingredients:

- 1 and ½ cups coconut flour
- 1 teaspoon baking powder
- ½ teaspoon vanilla extract
- 2 eggs, whisked
- 2 cups Greek yogurt
- ½ cup swerve
- 3 tablespoons coconut flakes
- 2 cups water

Directions:

In a bowl, mix the flour with the baking powder and the rest of the ingredients except the water, whisk well and pour into a pudding pan. Add the water to the instant pot, add the steamer basket, put the pudding pan inside, put the lid on and cook on High for 30 minutes. Release the pressure naturally for 10 minutes and serve the pudding cold.

Nutrition: calories 94, fat 4.3, fiber 0.4, carbs 1.5, protein 4.9

Pecans and Plums Bread

Preparation time: 10 minutes | Cooking time: 30 minutes | Servings: 4

Ingredients:

- 1 cup coconut flour
- 3 eggs, whisked
- 1 tablespoon vanilla extract
- 1 and ½ cups swerve
- 2 cups plums, pitted and chopped
- 2 cups coconut milk
- 2 tablespoons pecans, chopped
- ¼ teaspoon baking powder
- 2 cups water
- Cooking spray

Directions:

In a bowl, combine the coconut flour with the eggs and the rest of the ingredients except the cooking spray and the water and whisk well. Grease a loaf pan with the cooking spray and pour the bread mix inside. Add the water to the instant pot, add the steamer basket, put the loaf pan inside, put the lid on and cook on High for 30 minutes. Release the pressure naturally for 10 minutes, cool the bread down, slice and serve.

Nutrition: calories 348, fat 23.5, fiber 3.1, carbs 6.6, protein 7.2

Chocolate Cheesecake

Preparation time: 10 minutes | Cooking time: 40 minutes | Servings: 6

Ingredients:

- 2 tablespoons ghee, melted
- 1 cup heavy cream
- 2 ounces chocolate, melted
- ½ cup swerve
- 12 ounces cream cheese, soft
- 1 and ½ teaspoon vanilla extract
- 2 eggs, whisked
- Cooking spray
- 1 cup water

Directions:

Grease a spring form pan with cooking spray and leave it aside. In a bowl, mix the ghee with the chocolate, the cream and the rest of the ingredients except the water, whisk well and pour into the pan. Add the water to the instant pot, add the steamer basket, put the pan inside, put the lid on and cook on Low for 40 minutes. Release the pressure naturally for 10 minutes, and serve the cheesecake cold.

Nutrition: calories 282, fat 25.4, fiber 0.2, carbs 5.8, protein 5.5

Plums and Rice Pudding

Preparation time: 6 minutes | Cooking time: 20 minutes | Servings: 4

Ingredients:

- 2 cups coconut milk
- 1 cup cauliflower rice
- ½ cup plums, pitted and chopped
- ¼ cup heavy cream
- 2 eggs, whisked
- ½ cup swerve
- ½ teaspoon vanilla extract

Directions:

In your instant pot, mix the cauliflower rice with the plums and the rest of the ingredients, put the lid on and cook on High for 20 minutes. Release the pressure fast for 6 minutes, divide the pudding into bowls and serve cold.

Nutrition: calories 339, fat 27.7, fiber 2.7, carbs 6.5, protein 5.7

Cinnamon Berries Custard

Preparation time: 10 minutes | Cooking time: 15 minutes | Servings: 4

Ingredients:

- 3 eggs, whisked
- 2 cups coconut milk
- 1/3 cup swerve
- 1 tablespoon ghee, melted
- ½ cup heavy cream
- 1 tablespoon cinnamon powder
- ½ cup raspberries
- 1 teaspoon vanilla extract
- 1 and ½ cups water

Directions:

In a bowl, combine the eggs with the milk and the rest of the ingredients except the water, whisk well and transfer to a pan that fits the instant pot. Add the water to the instant pot, add the steamer basket, put the pan inside, put the lid on and cook on High for 15 minutes. Release the pressure naturally for 10 minutes, divide the mix in bowls and serve really cold.

Nutrition: calories 1276, fat 26.7, fiber 2.4, carbs 6.2, protein 4.9

Ginger and Cardamom Plums Mix

Preparation time: 10 minutes | Cooking time: 15 minutes | Servings: 4

Ingredients:

- 3 cups plums, pitted and halved
- 2 cups heavy cream
- 1 tablespoon ginger, grated
- 3 tablespoons swerve
- 2 teaspoons vanilla extract
- ¼ teaspoon cardamom, ground

Directions:

In your instant pot, combine the plums with the cream and the rest of the ingredients, put the lid on and cook on High for 15 minutes. Release the pressure naturally for 10 minutes, divide the mix into bowls and serve cold.

Nutrition: calories 241, fat 22.4, fiber 0.9, carbs 6, protein 1.7

Chocolate Cake
Preparation time: 10 minutes | Cooking time: 30 minutes | Servings: 4

Ingredients:
- 1 and ½ cups almond flour
- 1 cup cocoa powder
- Cooking spray
- 1 cup coconut flour
- 2 teaspoons baking powder
- 2 teaspoons baking soda
- ¼ cup flaxseed meal
- ½ cup ghee, melted
- 1 cup swerve
- 4 eggs, whisked
- 1 cup almond milk
- 1 teaspoon vanilla extract
- 2 cups water

Directions:
In a bowl, combine the almond flour with the cocoa, coconut flour and the rest of the ingredients except the cooking spray and the water and whisk really well. Grease a cake pan with the cooking spray and pour the cake mix inside. Add the water to the instant pot, put the steamer basket, add the cake pan inside, put the lid on and cook on High for 30 minutes. Release the pressure naturally for 10 minutes, cool the cake down, slice and serve.

Nutrition: calories 344, fat 33.1, fiber 3.4, carbs 5.8, protein 8.1

Chocolate Cookies
Preparation time: 10 minutes | Cooking time: 30 minutes | Servings: 4

Ingredients:
- 2 eggs, whisked
- ½ cup ghee, melted
- 2 tablespoons heavy cream
- 2 teaspoons vanilla extract
- 2 and ¾ cups almond flour
- ¼ cup swerve
- 1 cup chocolate chips
- Cooking spray
- 1 and ½ cups water

Directions:
In a bowl, mix the eggs with the ghee and the rest of the ingredients except the cooking spray and the water and whisk well. Put the water in the instant pot, add the steamer basket inside, arrange the cookies inside, spray them with cooking spray, put the lid on and cook on High for 30 minutes. Release the pressure naturally for 10 minutes, and serve the cookies cold.

Nutrition: calories 257, fat 21.4, fiber 0.7, carbs 12.5, protein 3.1

Coffee Cake
Preparation time: 10 minutes | Cooking time: 40 minutes | Servings: 4

Ingredients:
- 1/3 cup brewed coffee
- 1 and ½ cups almond flour
- ½ cup ghee, melted
- 1 and ½ cups swerve
- ½ teaspoon baking powder
- 4 eggs, whisked
- 1 teaspoon vanilla extract
- Cooking spray
- 1 cup water

Directions:
In a bowl, combine the coffee with the flour and the rest of the ingredients except the cooking spray and the water and whisk well. Grease a cake pan with the cooking spray and pour the cake mix inside. Put the water in the instant pot, add the steamer basket, put the cake pan inside, put the lid on and cook on High for 40 minutes. Release the pressure naturally for 10 minutes, cool the cake down, slice and serve.

Nutrition: calories 195, fat 20, fiber 0, carbs 0.5, protein 3.8

Nutmeg Pudding
Preparation time: 10 minutes | Cooking time: 30 minutes | Servings: 6

Ingredients:
- 2 cups water
- Cooking spray
- ½ cup swerve
- 4 eggs, whisked
- 1 cup heavy cream
- ½ cup almond flour
- 1 teaspoon nutmeg, ground
- ½ teaspoon baking soda
- 2/3 cup ghee, melted

Directions:
In a bowl, mix the swerve with the eggs and the rest of the ingredients except the cooking spray and the water and whisk._Grease a pudding pan with the cooking spray and pour the pudding mix inside._Put the water in the instant pot, add the steamer basket, put the pudding pan inside, put the lid on and cook on High for 30 minutes._Release the pressure naturally for 10 minutes, cool the pudding down and serve.

Nutrition: calories 235, fat 24.7, fiber 0.1, carbs 0.7, protein 3.2

Chocolate Chips Balls

Preparation time: 5 minutes | *Cooking time:* 6 minutes | *Servings:* 6

Ingredients:
- 1 cup chocolate chips
- 2 tablespoons ghee, melted
- 2/3 cup heavy cream
- 2 tablespoons swerve
- ¼ teaspoon vanilla extract
- 1 cup water

Directions:

In a bowl, combine the chocolate chips with the ghee and the rest of the ingredients except the water, stir well and shape medium balls out of this mix. Put the water in the instant pot, add the steamer basket, put the balls inside, put the lid on and cook on High for 6 minutes. Release the pressure fast for 5 minutes and serve the chocolate balls cold.

Nutrition: calories 350, fat 23.8, fiber 1.4, carbs 6.9, protein 3.6

Coconut and Cocoa Doughnuts

Preparation time: 10 minutes | *Cooking time:* 20 minutes | *Servings:* 4

Ingredients:
- ¼ cup swerve
- ¼ cup flaxseed meal
- ¾ cup coconut flour
- 1 teaspoon baking powder
- 1 teaspoon vanilla extract
- 2 eggs, whisked
- 3 tablespoons ghee, melted
- ¼ cup coconut milk
- 1 tablespoon cocoa powder
- Cooking spray
- 1 cup water

Directions:

In a bowl, mix the swerve with the flaxmeal and the rest of the ingredients except the cooking spray and the water and stir well. Grease a doughnut pan with the cooking spray and divide the mix. Add the water to the instant pot, add the steamer basket, put the pan inside, put the lid on and cook on High for 20 minutes. Release the pressure naturally for 10 minutes, cool the doughnuts down and serve.

Nutrition: calories 196, fat 17.3, fiber 2.7, carbs 4.5, protein 4.7

Chocolate Balls

Preparation time: 5 minutes | Cooking time: 10 minutes | Servings: 10

Ingredients:

- 1 cup ghee, melted
- 3 tablespoons macadamia nuts, chopped
- ¼ cup stevia
- 5 tablespoons unsweetened coconut powder
- 2 tablespoons cocoa powder
- 1 cup water

Directions:

In a bowl, combine the ghee with the macadamia nuts and the rest of the ingredients except the water, whisk really well and shape medium balls out of this mix. Add the water to the instant pot, add the steamer basket, arrange the balls inside, put the lid on and cook on High for 10 minutes. Release the pressure fast for 5 minutes and serve the balls cold.

Nutrition: calories 200, fat 22.4, fiber 0.5, carbs 0.9, protein 0.5

Vanilla and Cocoa Cream

Preparation time: 5 minutes | Cooking time: 5 minutes | Servings: 4

Ingredients:

- 1 and ½ cups heavy cream
- 3 tablespoons swerve
- 2 tablespoons cocoa powder
- 1 teaspoon vanilla extract
- 1 and ½ cups water

Directions:

In a bowl, combine the heavy cream with the rest of the ingredients except the water, whisk well and divide into 4 ramekins. Put the water in the instant pot, add the steamer basket, put the ramekins inside, put the lid on and cook on High for 5 minutes. Release the pressure fast for 5 minutes and serve the cream cold.

Nutrition: calories 216, fat 22.6, fiber 0.8, carbs 3.3, protein 1.7

Plums Pie

Preparation time: 10 minutes | Cooking time: 30 minutes | Servings: 8

Ingredients:
For the crust:
- 1 cup coconut, unsweetened and shredded
- 1 cup pecans, chopped

- ¼ cup ghee, melted

For the filling:
- 8 ounces cream cheese
- 4 ounces strawberries
- 2 tablespoons water
- ½ tablespoon lime juice

- 1 teaspoon swerve
- ½ cup heavy cream
- 1 and ½ cups water

Directions:
In a bowl, combine the coconut with the pecans and the ghee, stir well and press on the bottom of a lined pie pan. In a second bowl, combine the cream cheese with the rest of the ingredients except the water, whisk well, pour over the crust and spread well. Add the water to the instant pot, add the steamer basket, put the pie pan inside, put the lid on and cook on High for 30 minutes. Release the pressure naturally for 10 minutes, cool the pie down, slice and serve.

Nutrition: calories 221, fat 22.4, fiber 1.2, carbs 3.6, protein 2.8

Vanilla Cream Mix

Preparation time: 10 minutes | Cooking time: 20 minutes | Servings: 4

Ingredients:
- 1 tablespoon vanilla extract
- 4 tablespoons butter
- 4 tablespoons sour cream
- 16 ounces cream cheese, soft

- ½ cup swerve
- ½ cup cocoa powder
- 1 cup heavy cream
- 2 cups water

Directions:
In a bowl, combine the vanilla with the butter and the rest of the ingredients except the water, whisk well and divide into 4 ramekins. Add the water to the instant pot, add the steamer basket, put the ramekins inside, put the lid on and cook on High for 20 minutes. Release the pressure naturally for 10 minutes, and serve the cream cold.

Nutrition: calories 330, fat 20.2, fiber 1.6, carbs 5.4, protein 5.8

Mascarpone Cheesecake

Preparation time: 5 minutes | Cooking time: 15 minutes | Servings: 6

Ingredients:

- 2 tablespoons butter, soft
- 1 cup heavy cream
- 2 ounces chocolate, melted
- ½ cup swerve
- 12 ounces mascarpone cheese
- 1 and ½ teaspoon cocoa powder
- 1 egg, whisked
- Cooking spray
- 1 cup water

Directions:

In a bowl, combine the butter with the cream and the rest of the ingredients except the cooking spray and the water and whisk well. Grease a cake pan with the cooking spray and pour the mix inside. Add the water to the instant pot, add the steamer basket, put the cake pan inside, put the lid on and cook on High for 15 minutes. Release the pressure fast for 5 minutes, cool the cheesecake down and serve.

Nutrition: calories 263, fat 22.2, fiber 0.3, carbs 6, protein 8.5

Creamy Chocolate Avocado Mix

Preparation time: 5 minutes | Cooking time: 5 minutes | Servings: 4

Ingredients:

- 2 avocados, peeled, pitted and chopped
- 1 cup heavy cream
- ½ cup chocolate chips
- ¼ cup swerve
- 1 teaspoon vanilla extract
- 1 cup water

Directions:

In your food processor, combine the avocados with the rest of the ingredients except the water, pulse well and divide into 4 ramekins. Put the water in the instant pot, add the steamer basket, put the ramekins inside, put the lid on and cook on High for 5 minutes. Release the pressure fast for 5 minutes, and serve the creamy mix really cold.

Nutrition: calories 283, fat 24.6, fiber 4, carbs 4.8, protein 2.8

Vanilla Chocolate Cupcakes

Preparation time: 10 minutes | Cooking time: 20 minutes | Servings: 12

Ingredients:
- ½ cup butter, melted
- ½ cup avocado oil
- ½ cup coconut, shredded
- 2 ounces chocolate, chopped
- ¼ cup cocoa powder
- ¼ teaspoon vanilla extract
- ¼ cup swerve
- 1 cup water

Directions:

In a bowl, combine the butter with the oil and the rest of the ingredients except the water and whisk really well. Line a cupcake pan that fits the instant pot with parchment paper and divide the chocolate mix inside. Put the water in the instant pot, add the steamer basket, add the cupcake pan inside, put the lid on and cook on High for 20 minutes. Release the pressure naturally for 10 minutes and serve the cupcakes cold.

Nutrition: calories 243, fat 23.2, fiber 2.7, carbs 6.8, protein 2

Cream Cheese and Blackberries Mousse

Preparation time: 4 minutes | Cooking time: 4 minutes | Servings: 4

Ingredients:
- 8 ounces cream cheese
- 1 teaspoon serve
- 1 cup heavy cream
- 1 tablespoon blackberries
- 1 cup water

Directions:

In a bowl, mix the cream with the other ingredients except the water, whisk well and divide into 2 ramekins. Put the water in the instant pot, add the steamer basket, put the ramekins inside, put the lid on and cook on High for 4 minutes. Release the pressure fast for 4 minutes and serve the mousse really cold.

Nutrition: calories 202, fat 20.5, fiber 0.1, carbs 1.7, protein 3.3

Conclusion

The instant pot is such an innovative and futuristic cooking tool. It has gained so many fans all over the world. The instant pot allows you to cook delicious meals for all your family in a matter of minutes and with minimum effort. The best thing about the instant pot is that you don't need to be an expert cook to make tasty culinary feasts. You just need the right ingredients and the correct directions. That's how you'll get the best instant pot meals.

This great culinary guide you've just discovered is more than a simple instant pot cooking journal. It is a Ketogenic instant pot recipes collection you will find very useful.
The Ketogenic diet will give you the energy boost you need, it will make you lose the extra weight and it will improve your overall health in a matter of days. This collection contains the best Ketogenic instant pot dishes you can prepare in the comfort of your own home. All these dishes are so flavored and textured and they all taste incredible.

So, if you are following a Ketogenic diet and you own an instant pot, get your own copy of this cookbook and start your Ketogenic culinary adventure. Cook the best Ketogenic instant pot meals and enjoy them all!

Recipe Index

236

BELL PEPPER (YELLOW)
Bell Peppers and Cauliflower Salad, 16
Turkey Bowls, 33
Mixed Peppers and Parsley, 214
Saffron Bell Peppers, 78
Marinated Turkey Mix, 165

BLACKBERRIES
Blackberry Muffins, 14
Sweet Berries Bowls, 35
Turkey and Blackberries Sauce, 163
Vanilla Blackberries Bowls, 216
Berry Chocolate Cream, 217
Berries and Nuts Pudding, 221
Macadamia Blackberry Stew, 223
Cream Cheese and Blackberries Mousse, 234

BLUEBERRIES
Coconut Blueberry Pudding, 19
Chia and Blueberries Bowls, 22
Creamy Blueberries and Nuts, 29
Berries and Nuts Pudding, 221
Plums and Berries Compote, 223

BOK CHOY
Ginger Cauliflower Rice Pudding, 25
Kale and Bok Choy Muffins, 30
Zucchinis and Bok Choy, 79
Beef, Sprouts and Bok Choy Mix, 177
Pork and Bok Choy, 194
Lemon Peppers and Bok Choy, 209
Tomato Bok Choy Mix, 210
Balsamic Bok Choy and Onions, 211
Bok Choy and Parmesan Mix, 212
Ginger Cauliflower Rice Pudding, 25

BROCCOLI
Chives Broccoli Mash, 75
Broccoli Casserole, 15
Scallions and Broccoli Mix, 17
Avocado and Broccoli Salad, 18
Broccoli and Cheese Pancake, 20
Broccoli and Almonds Mix, 37
Curry Cauliflower Rice Bowls, 39
Broccoli and Zucchini Soup, 50
Mozzarella Broccoli, 65
Garlic Broccoli Mix, 65
Celery and Broccoli Mix, 73
Broccoli Dip, 91
Cod and Broccoli, 116
Sage Chicken and Broccoli, 145
Marinated Turkey Mix, 165
Lamb and Broccoli Mix, 178
Broccoli and Watercress Mix, 211
Lemon and Pesto Broccoli, 212

BRUSSELS SPROUTS
Chicken and Brussels Sprouts Stew, 59
Creamy Brussels Sprouts Stew, 63
Chives Brussels Sprouts, 64
Thyme Brussels Sprouts, 75
Lemon Brussels Sprouts and Tomatoes, 77
Halibut and Brussels Sprouts, 140
Tomato Turkey and Sprouts, 144
Chicken Casserole, 160
Chicken and Green Sauté, 161
Chicken and Green Sauté, 161
Turkey, Brussels Sprouts and Walnuts, 167
Beef, Sprouts and Bok Choy Mix, 177
Spicy Beef, Sprouts and Avocado Mix, 192
Coconut Leeks and Sprouts, 198
Brussels Sprouts and Sauce, 201
Bell Peppers and Brussels Sprouts, 202
Dill Fennel and Brussels Sprouts, 207
Buttery Turmeric Brussels Sprouts, 212

BUTTER
Vanilla Cream Mix, 232
Mascarpone Cheesecake, 233
Vanilla Chocolate Cupcakes, 234

CABBAGE
Ginger Cabbage and Radish Mix, 64

CABBAGE (GREEN)
Cabbage Soup, 52
Turmeric Cabbage Stew, 57
Lemon Cabbage Mix, 69
Cabbage and Tomatoes, 83
Leeks and Cabbage, 86
Eggplants and Cabbage Mix, 209
Cabbage and Peppers, 78

CABBAGE (RED)
Cabbage and Spinach Slaw, 109
Turkey and Cabbage Mix, 145
Tarragon Chicken Mix, 147
Chicken, Cabbage and Leeks, 150
Mustard Greens and Cabbage Sauté, 205
Garlic Cabbage and Watercress, 210
Balsamic and Coconut Cabbage, 211
Red Cabbage and Artichokes, 80
Cabbage, Tomato and Avocado Salsa, 110
Cilantro Red Cabbage and Artichokes, 207

CABBAGE (SAVOY)
Pine Nuts Savoy Cabbage, 70
Beef and Savoy Cabbage Mix, 196
Balsamic Savoy Cabbage, 207

Coconut Blueberry Pudding, 19
Coconut Yogurt Mix, 23
Coconut Pudding, 32
Coconut Oatmeal, 36
Coconut Omelet, 3
Okra Soup, 42
Bacon Artichokes, 82
Creamy Catfish, 140
Cheddar Turkey, 166
Almond Lamb Meatloaf, 194
Coconut Zucchini Cake, 216
Cantaloupe Pudding, 218
Coconut Raspberries Bowls, 218
Zucchini Rice Pudding, 220
Berries and Nuts Pudding, 221
Chocolate and Brazil Nuts Bread, 225
Pecans and Plums Bread, 226
Plums and Rice Pudding, 227
Cinnamon Berries Custard, 227
Coconut and Cocoa Doughnuts, 230
Cinnamon Turkey Curry, 46

COD
Cod and Basil Tomato Passata, 134
Cod and Tomato Passata, 47
Hot Cod Stew, 54
Cod and Shrimp Stew, 59
Salmon and Cod Cakes, 94
Green Beans and Cod Salad, 94
Cod and Tomatoes, 113
Cod and Cilantro Sauce, 113
Coriander Cod Mix, 114
Cod and Zucchinis, 115
Cod and Broccoli, 116
Cinnamon Cod Mix, 117
Saffron Chili Cod, 121
Lime Cod Mix, 131
Cod and Asparagus, 133
Smoked Crab and Cod Mix, 136

CRAB
Thyme Crab and Spinach, 136
Smoked Crab and Cod Mix, 136
Crab, Spinach and Chives, 137

CRANBERRIES
Cranberries Cauliflower Rice, 87

CREAM
Broccoli Casserole, 15
Creamy Eggs Ramekins, 18
Chili Frittata, 21
Parsley Cauliflower Mix, 24
Pork Pie, 24
Creamy Zucchini Pan, 28

Zucchini Spread, 32
Broccoli and Almonds Mix, 37
Salmon and Dill Sauce, 126
Haddock and Cilantro Sauce, 130
White Duck Chili, 157
Creamy Chicken Wings, 163
Tuscan Chicken, 164
Creamy Asparagus Mix, 200
Brussels Sprouts and Sauce, 201
Cayenne Peppers and Sauce, 202
Creamy Eggplant Mix, 204
Creamy Okra and Collard Greens, 206
Berry Chocolate Cream, 217
Watermelon Cream, 218
Egg and Cantaloupe Pudding, 219
Creamy Rice Pudding, 220
Heavy Cream and Raspberries Ramekins, 224
Chocolate Cheesecake, 226
Plums and Rice Pudding, 227
Cinnamon Berries Custard, 227
Ginger and Cardamom Plums Mix, 227
Chocolate Cookies, 228
Nutmeg Pudding, 229
Chocolate Chips Balls, 230
Vanilla and Cocoa Cream, 231
Plums Pie, 232
Vanilla Cream Mix, 232
Mascarpone Cheesecake, 233
Creamy Chocolate Avocado Mix, 233
Cream Cheese and Blackberries Mousse, 234

CREAM CHEESE
Creamy Eggs Ramekins, 18
Zucchini Spread, 32
Creamy Green Beans, 69
Cheesy Radish Spread, 112
Creamy Rice Pudding, 220
Chocolate Cheesecake, 226
Plums Pie, 232
Vanilla Cream Mix, 232
Cream Cheese and Blackberries Mousse, 234

CUCUMBERS
Egg Salad, 40
Oregano Green Beans Salsa, 88
Eggplants, Cucumber and Olives, 209

DATES
Oregano Chicken and Dates, 157

DUCK
Duck and Fennel, 147
Duck and Hot Eggplant Mix, 149
Duck and Coriander Sauce, 152
Duck, Leeks and Asparagus, 155

Lime Cherry Bowls, 220
Lime Coconut Vanilla Cream, 221
Raspberries and Coconut Puddings, 222
Cabbage and Peppers, 78
Salmon and Cod Cakes, 94
Parsley Clams Platter, 97
Oregano Beef Bites, 105
Lime Glazed Salmon, 129
Salmon and Coconut Mix, 130
Lime Cod Mix, 131
Turkey and Lime Dill Sauce, 148
Lime and Paprika Asparagus, 198
Buttery Turmeric Brussels Sprouts, 212
Cinnamon Cream, 222

LIME JUICE
Lime Pork Bowls, 43
Cod and Tomato Passata, 47
Artichokes Cream, 61
Garlic Broccoli Mix, 65
Collard Greens and Tomatoes, 66
Celery and Broccoli Mix, 73
Green Beans and Cod Salad, 94
Parsley Clams Platter, 97
Olives and Spinach Dip, 106
Red Chard Spread, 107
Salmon and Swiss Chard Salad, 108
Lime Shrimp, 116
Catfish and Avocado Mix, 127
Lime Glazed Salmon, 129
Salmon and Coconut Mix, 130
Lime Cod Mix, 131
Chipotle Tilapia Mix, 139
Creamy Catfish, 140
Duck and Fennel, 147
Lime and Paprika Asparagus, 198
Okra and Olives Mix, 208
Lime Cherry Bowls, 220
Cinnamon Cream, 222
Lime Watermelon Compote, 224
Greek Turkey and Sauce, 42
Basil Shrimp and Eggplants, 46
Cabbage and Peppers, 78
Mint Zucchinis, 87
Lime Spinach and Leeks Dip, 89
Balsamic Endives, 100
Thyme Eggplants and Celery Spread, 101
Oregano Beef Bites, 105
Basil Peppers Salsa, 108
Coriander Cod Mix, 114
Sea Bass and Sauce, 119
Rosemary Tilapia and Pine Nuts, 137
Turkey and Lime Dill Sauce, 148
Marinated Turkey Mix, 165
Lime Pork Chops, 180

Beef and Endives Mix, 183
Mint Lamb Chops, 185
Hot Curry Lamb and Green Beans, 187
Tomato Bok Choy Mix, 210
Lime Coconut Vanilla Cream, 221
Macadamia Blackberry Stew, 223
Plums Pie, 232

MACKEREL
Mackerel and Shrimp Mix, 122
Mackerel and Basil Sauce, 122

MUSHROOMS
Mushroom and Chicken Soup, 47
Chili Mushrooms Stew, 57
Cheesy Mushroom and Tomato Salad, 103

MUSHROOMS (BROWN)
Herbed Mushroom Mix, 27

MUSHROOMS (WHITE)
Mushroom and Avocado Salad, 26
Mushroom and Okra Omelet, 36
Mushroom and Cauliflower Rice Salad, 37
Pork Chops and Thyme Mushrooms, 44
Balsamic Mushroom and Radish Mix, 66
Paprika Mushrooms, 67
Chard and Mushrooms Mix, 68
Mushrooms and Endives Mix, 74
Parmesan Mushroom Spread, 90
Mushrooms Salsa, 102
Chicken and Balsamic Mushrooms, 151
Chicken, Peppers and Mushrooms, 166
Beef and Mushroom Rice, 183

MUSSELS
Balsamic Mussels Bowls, 95
Mussels Salad, 104
Shrimp and Mussels Salad, 110

MUSTARD (GREENS)
Mustard Greens Dip, 92
Tuna and Mustard Greens, 120
Chicken and Green Sauté, 161
Chicken and Green Sauté, 161
Mustard Greens and Cabbage Sauté, 205

NUTMEG
Sweet Zucchini Mix, 34
Strawberries and Nuts Salad, 35
Spinach and Fennel Mix, 71
Zucchini Mix, 74
Spinach and Kale Mix, 76
Creamy Fennel, 77
Bacon Artichokes, 82

PECANS
Strawberries and Pecans Cream, 217
Berries and Nuts Pudding, 221
Coconut Pecans Cream, 224
Pecans and Plums Bread, 226
Plums Pie, 232

PEPPER (CAYENNE)
Cayenne Pork and Artichokes Stew, 49
Kale Stew, 56
Cabbage and Tomatoes, 83
Chili Cauliflower Rice, 85
Basil Spicy Artichokes, 198
Cayenne Peppers and Sauce, 202

PEPPER (CHILI)
Mushroom and Okra Omelet, 36
Balsamic Mussels Bowls, 95
Mackerel and Basil Sauce, 122
Ginger Cauliflower Spread, 91
Asparagus and Eggs Mix, 22
Cinnamon Turkey Curry, 46
Cayenne Pork and Artichokes Stew, 49
Chili Tomato and Zucchini Dip, 90

PEPPER (LEMON)
Salmon and Dill Sauce, 126

PEPPER CHILI (GREEN)
Mint Lamb Chops, 185

PEPPER FLAKES (RED)
Bell Pepper Cream, 53
Tomato and Zucchini Salsa, 96
Shrimp and Beef Bowls, 98
Mackerel and Basil Sauce, 122
Spicy Tilapia and Kale, 128
Turkey and Hot Lemon Sauce, 156
Spicy Pork, Zucchinis and Eggplants, 172
Pork Meatballs and Spring Onions Sauce, 173
Italian Leg of Lamb, 186
Pork and Bok Choy, 194
Basil Spicy Artichokes, 198
Balsamic Bok Choy and Onions, 211
Lemon Tomato and Green Beans, 214

PINE NUTS
Pine Nuts Savoy Cabbage, 70
Sea Bass and Pesto, 120
Rosemary Tilapia and Pine Nuts, 137
Pine Nuts Lamb Meatballs, 189

PLUMS
Plums and Raisins Mix, 216
Lime Coconut Vanilla Cream, 221

Plums and Berries Compote, 223
Pecans and Plums Bread, 226
Plums and Rice Pudding, 227
Ginger and Cardamom Plums Mix, 227
Lime Coconut Vanilla Cream, 221

POMEGRANATE
Coconut Oatmeal, 36

PORK
Scotch Eggs and Tomato Passata, 23
Leeks and Pork Mix, 28
Pork Meatballs and Spring Onions Sauce, 173
Pork Hash, 17
Pork Pie, 24
Pork and Kale Hash, 34
Lime Pork Bowls, 43
Pork Chops and Thyme Mushrooms, 44
Mexican Pork and Okra Salad, 44
Pork and Kale Meatballs, 45
Pork and Baby Spinach, 45
Tomato and Pork Soup, 48
Cayenne Pork and Artichokes Stew, 49
Garlic and Parsley Pork, 168
Rosemary and Cinnamon Pork, 168
Curry Pork and Kale, 169
Pork and Cilantro Tomato Mix, 169
Mustard Pork and Chard, 170
Pork, Spinach and Green Beans, 170
Pork, Kale and Capers Mix, 171
Pork and Lemon Basil Sauce, 171
Pork and Cauliflower Rice, 172
Spicy Pork, Zucchinis and Eggplants, 172
Raspberry Pork Mix, 173
Chili Pork Chops, 174
Rosemary Pork Chops, 174
Pork Chops and Green Chilies Mix, 175
Sage and Tarragon Pork, 175
Coconut Pork Mix, 176
Coriander Beef and Pork Mix, 179
Pork Ribs and Green Beans, 180
Lime Pork Chops, 180
Pesto Pork and Mustard Greens, 181
Pork and Olives, 182
Spinach Pork Meatloaf, 190
Pork and Chives Asparagus, 193
Pork and Bok Choy, 194
Pork and Mint Zucchinis, 196

RADISHES
Ginger Cabbage and Radish Mix, 64
Cheesy Tomato and Radish Salad, 33
Balsamic Mushroom and Radish Mix, 66
Spinach and Radish Mix, 69
Radish Salsa, 92

251

Pork and Olives, 182
Feta Cheese Lamb Mix, 184
Mustard and Sage Beef, 184
Spiced Lamb Meatballs, 185
Herbed Crusted Lamb Cutlets, 188
Spinach Pork Meatloaf, 190
Ginger Lamb and Basil, 191
Beef and Savoy Cabbage Mix, 196
Beef and Walnuts Rice, 197
Mustard Greens and Cabbage Sauté, 205
Dill Zucchini, Tomatoes and Eggplants, 206
Cilantro Red Cabbage and Artichokes, 207
Dill Fennel and Brussels Sprouts, 207
Okra and Olives Mix, 208
Broccoli and Watercress Mix, 211
Bok Choy and Parmesan Mix, 212

TOMATO PASTE
Bell Pepper Cream, 53
Chicken and Brussels Sprouts Stew, 59
Leek Soup, 62
Sage Chicken and Turkey Stew, 62
Spiced Chicken Bites, 141
Duck and Hot Eggplant Mix, 149
Spicy Pork, Zucchinis and Eggplants, 172

TOMATOES
Soft Eggs and Avocado Mix, 14
Turkey Omelet, 34
Watercress and Zucchini Salsa, 105
Turkey and Cabbage Mix, 145
Ginger Cauliflower Rice Pudding, 25
Chicken Bowls, 31
Curry Cauliflower Rice Bowls, 39
Cinnamon Turkey Curry, 46
Tomato and Pork Soup, 48
Green Beans Soup, 49
Curry Tomato Cream, 51
Eggplant Soup, 53
Bell Pepper Cream, 53
Lamb Stew, 55
Shrimp and Olives Stew, 55
Turkey Stew, 56
Salmon Stew, 60
Veggie Soup, 61
Sage Chicken and Turkey Stew, 62
Tomato and Olives Stew, 63
Oregano Green Beans Salsa, 88
Chili Tomato and Zucchini Dip, 90
Radish Salsa, 92
Tomato and Zucchini Salsa, 96
Mushrooms Salsa, 102
Cheesy Mushroom and Tomato Salad, 103
Basil Peppers Salsa, 108
Pesto Chicken Salad, 109

Beef, Arugula and Olives Salad, 111
Cod and Tomatoes, 113
Salmon and Salsa, 121
Oregano Tuna, 123
Tilapia Salad, 125
Haddock and Cilantro Sauce, 130
Thyme Crab and Spinach, 136
Chili Haddock and Tomatoes, 138
Ginger Halibut, 139
Tarragon Chicken Mix, 147
Turkey and Cilantro Tomato Salsa, 161
Beef, Cauliflower Rice and Shrimp Mix, 176
Paprika Lamb Chops, 181
Lamb and Sun-dried Tomatoes Mix, 187
Smoked Paprika Lamb, 195
Cheddar Tomatoes, 203
Tomato and Dill Sauté, 205
Dill Zucchini, Tomatoes and Eggplants, 206

TOMATOES (CANNED)
Cayenne Pork and Artichokes Stew, 49
Kale Stew, 56
Turmeric Cabbage Stew, 57
Beef and Cauliflower Stew, 58
Cod and Shrimp Stew, 59
Spicy Tilapia and Kale, 128
Cod and Basil Tomato Passata, 134
Pine Nuts Lamb Meatballs, 189
Lemon Tomato and Green Beans, 214
Tilapia and Red Sauce, 131

TOMATOES (CHERRY)
Tomato and Peppers Salad, 20
Tomato and Zucchini Salad, 32
Cheesy Tomato and Radish Salad, 33
Collard Greens and Tomatoes, 66
Dill Cherry Tomatoes, 71
Tomatoes and Cauliflower Mix, 71
Thyme Tomatoes, 76
Lemon Brussels Sprouts and Tomatoes, 77
Cabbage and Tomatoes, 83
Artichokes and Salmon Bowls, 93
Cabbage, Tomato and Avocado Salsa, 110
Cinnamon Cod Mix, 117
Tuscan Chicken, 164
Lamb Chops, Fennel and Tomatoes, 186
Asparagus and Tomatoes, 199
Creamy Tomatoes, 204
Tomato Bok Choy Mix, 210

TROUT
Paprika Trout, 115
Trout and Radishes, 116
Rosemary Trout and Cauliflower, 117
Trout and Eggplant Mix, 118

Made in the USA
San Bernardino, CA
26 November 2019

60235271R00158